Critical Perspectives on Coercive Interventions

Coercive medico-legal interventions are often employed to prevent people deemed to be unable to make competent decisions about their health, such as minors, people with mental illness, disability or problematic alcohol or other drug use, from harming themselves or others. These interventions can entail major curtailments of individuals' liberty and bodily integrity, and may cause significant harm and distress.

Examining the ethical, social and legal issues involved in coerced care, this book brings together the views and insights of leading researchers from a range of disciplines, including criminology, law, ethics, psychology and public health, as well as legal and medical practitioners, social-service 'consumers' and government officials. These contributions attempt to shed light on why we use coercive interventions, whether we should, whether they are effective in achieving the benefits that are offered to justify their use, and the impact that they have on some of society's most vulnerable citizens in the names of 'justice' and 'treatment'.

This book is essential reading for clinicians, researchers and legal practitioners involved in the study and application of coerced care, as well as students and scholars in the fields of law, medicine, ethics and criminology.

Claire Spivakovsky is a Senior Lecturer in Criminology at Monash University.

Kate Seear is an Associate Professor in Law at Monash University, an Australian Research Council DECRA Fellow, a practising lawyer, and an Adjunct Research Fellow at the National Drug Research Institute, Curtin University.

Adrian Carter is an NHMRC Career Development Fellow at the Monash Institute of Cognitive and Clinical Neurosciences and the School of Psychological Sciences, Monash University.

Routledge Frontiers of Criminal Justice

For more information about this series, please visit: https://www.routledge.com/Routledge-Frontiers-of-Criminal-Justice/book-series/RFCJ

Critical Perspectives on Coercive Interventions

Law, Medicine and Society

Edited by
Claire Spivakovsky, Kate Seear and
Adrian Carter

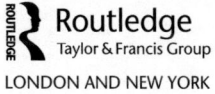

Routledge
Taylor & Francis Group

LONDON AND NEW YORK

First published 2018
by Routledge
2 Park Square, Milton Park, Abingdon, Oxon OX14 4RN

and by Routledge
711 Third Avenue, New York, NY 10017

Routledge is an imprint of the Taylor & Francis Group, an informa business

First issued in paperback 2020

British Library Cataloguing in Publication Data
A catalogue record for this book is available from the British Library

Library of Congress Cataloging in Publication Data
Names: Spivakovsky, Claire, editor.
Title: Critical perspectives on coercive interventions : law, medicine and
    society / edited by Claire Spivakovsky, Kate Seear and Adrian Carter.
Description: Milton Park, Abingdon, Oxon ; New York, NY : Routledge, 2018. |
    Series: Routledge frontiers of criminal justice ; 55 | Includes bibliographical
    references and index.
Identifiers: LCCN 2017052179| ISBN 9781138067370 (hbk) |
    ISBN 9781315158693 (ebk)
Subjects: LCSH: Involuntary treatment–Moral and ethical aspects. | Medical
    ethics–Miscellanea.
Classification: LCC R727.35 .C75 2018 | DDC 174.2–dc23
LC record available at https://lccn.loc.gov/2017052179

ISBN: 9781138067370 (hbk)
ISBN: 9780367482442 (pbk)
ISBN: 9781315158693 (ebk)

Typeset in Times New Roman
by Taylor & Francis Books

Contents

Boxes

Contributors

Robert Batey is Professorial Fellow, Flinders University and Senior Staff Specialist, Department of Medicine, Alice Springs Hospital. He has been engaged in Addiction Medical practice for 36 years and in Hepatology for 45 years. He continues an active research interest in alcohol related brain injury and in viral hepatitis. He was Clinical Advisor to NSW Health during the planning of the new Involuntary Treatment units established to function with the ending of the Inebriates Act of NSW.

Lisa Brophy is an Associate Professor with the University of Melbourne and Mind Australia's Principal Research Fellow. She has a career-long commitment to mental health through social work, research and teaching. Her research focus is on people experiencing mental illness and psychosocial disability and their recovery, social inclusion and human rights.

Adrian Carter is an Associate Professor and NHMRC Career Development Fellow and Head, Neuroscience and Society Group, School of Psychological Sciences, Monash Institute of Cognitive and Clinical Neurosciences, Monash University. He is also Director, Neuroethics Program, ARC Centre of Excellence for Integrative Brain Function and Chair, Australian Brain Alliance Neuroethics Subcommittee, Australian Academy of Science. His research examines the impact of neuroscience on our understanding and treatment of addiction and other compulsive behaviours. Associate Professor Carter has been an advisor to the WHO, the European Monitoring Centre for Drugs and Drug Addiction, and United Nations Office on Drugs and Crime.

John Chesterman is Director of Strategy at the Office of the Public Advocate. Dr Chesterman is a trained lawyer and prior to joining OPA he lectured in politics for more than eight years at the University of Melbourne. He has written a number of books, including (as co-author) *The Politics of Human Rights in Australia* (Cambridge University Press). In 2013 he travelled as a Churchill Fellow to the US, Canada and the UK, where he examined a variety of adult protection systems.

Ian Freckelton is a Queen's Counsel in full-time practice throughout Australia. He is also a Professorial Fellow of Law and Psychiatry and the Co-Director of the Master of Health Law programme at the University of Melbourne and an Adjunct Professor of Forensic Medicine at Monash University. Ian is the Editor of the *Journal of Law and Medicine* and the Editor-in-Chief of *Psychiatry, Psychology and Law.* He is a member of Victoria's Mental Health Tribunal and Coronial Council. He has written many books and articles on medical law and is a judge of the Supreme Court of Nauru.

Eleanore Fritze is a senior lawyer in Victoria Legal Aid's Mental Health & Disability Law program, where she advises and advocates before courts and tribunals on behalf of people subject to detention, compulsory treatment and other restrictions on their rights under Victoria's mental health and disability laws. Eleanore has a longstanding commitment to assisting people with mental illness and cognitive disabilities to access and meaningfully participate in the justice system and has received numerous awards for her studies and work, including a 2014 Churchill fellowship. She has previously worked as a personal carer and has also completed post-graduate disability studies.

Stephen Gray is a Senior Lecturer at Monash University Faculty of Law, and an Associate to the Castan Centre for Human Rights. He has published widely on Indigenous legal issues, including the Stolen Wages issue, criminal law, and protection for Indigenous art and culture. He was head researcher on the Northern Territory Intervention website, released by the Castan Centre for Human Rights in February 2016.

Wayne Hall is a Professor at the Centre for Youth Substance Abuse Research at the University of Queensland and at the National Addiction Centre, Kings College London. He has advised the World Health Organization on: the health effects of cannabis use; the effectiveness of drug substitution treatment; the contribution of illicit drug use to the global burden of disease; and the ethical implications of genetic and neuroscience research on addiction.

Bernadette McSherry, is the Foundation Director of the Melbourne Social Equity Institute at the University of Melbourne and an Adjunct Professor of Law in the Melbourne Law School and the Faculty of Law, Monash University. Professor McSherry is President of the Australian and New Zealand Association of Psychiatry, Psychology and Law and a legal member of the Mental Health Tribunal of Victoria. She became an Australian Research Council Federation Fellow in December 2007 and is a Fellow of the Academy of Social Sciences in Australia and a Fellow of the Australian Academy of Law.

Cath Roper has held a pioneering consumer academic role at the Centre for Psychiatric Nursing, University of Melbourne since 1999. Cath engages in policy development, promoting consumer perspective scholarship and co-designing consumer workforce innovations. She co-produces training in the specialist mental health service sector and teaches a consumer perspective subject to post-graduate mental health nurses. Cath experienced annual compulsory admissions to mental health services over 13 years, influencing her research interests, which include: understanding the impact of legislated contexts for consumers and clinicians, promoting practices supporting consumer self-determination and fostering consumer perspective as a unique discipline in the field of mental health.

Christopher James Ryan is a Clinical Associate Professor with the University of Sydney and Director of Consultation-Liaison Psychiatry at Sydney's Westmead Hospital. Though his work is primarily clinical, he maintains an active research programme. Many of his numerous publications focus on the interface of psychiatry, the law and human rights.

Kate Seear is an Associate Professor in Law at Monash University. She is the holder of a prestigious Australian Research Council DECRA fellowship. Through her DECRA fellowship she examines how the law conceptualises alcohol and other drug 'addiction'. Kate is also a practising lawyer and the Academic Director of Springvale Monash Legal Service. She is also an Adjunct Research Fellow at the National Drug Research Institute, Curtin University, Australia. Her research combines insights from feminist and social theory, science and technology studies, legal ethics and human rights.

Claire Spivakovsky is a Senior Lecturer in Criminology at Monash University. Dr Spivakovsky's work examines how the treatment of people with disability in society shapes the operation of norms, the power dynamics of normalisation and the experiences of that which we have come to think of as freedom. Dr Spivakovsky follows this research interest across a wide spectrum of topics, from the inclusive education of children with disability, to the everyday practices of disability group homes and the development of specialist mental health court procedures.

Linda Steele is a Senior Lecturer in the Faculty of Law at University of Technology Sydney and a Visiting Senior Fellow in the Faculty of Law, Humanities and the Arts at University of Wollongong. Linda's research explores the intersections of disability, law and injustice, with current projects focused on institutional violence, reproductive and sexual health, punishment and sexual violence. Linda has co-edited special issues of *Griffith Law Review, Continuum: Journal of Media & Cultural Studies, Australian Feminist Studies* and *Law in Context*. She is currently working on a monograph (under contract with Routledge's Social Justice Series) that provides a critical analysis of court diversion of people with disability.

Jamie Walvisch is a Lecturer at the Faculty of Law, Monash University. He has previously worked at the Judicial College of Victoria, the Australian Institute of Criminology and the Victorian Law Reform Commission. He has co-authored law reform reports on a wide range of topics, including defences to homicide, fraud and electronic commerce-related crime and road rage. His current research focuses on the intersection between law and psychiatry, especially in the sentencing context. He has published articles on this issue in leading journals, and has given presentations about it at numerous national and international conferences.

Penelope Weller is Director of the Juris Doctor Program in the Graduate School of Business and Law at RMIT University. Associate Professor Weller is a health and mental health law scholar and an internationally recognised expert on the Convention on the Rights of People with Disabilities. Weller teaches Administrative Law, Human Rights Law, Jurisprudence and Innovative Justice at RMIT. She is Chair of the College of Business Human Research Ethics Advisory Network and Deputy Chair of the University Human Research Ethics Committee at RMIT. She is a Community Member of the Mental Health Review Tribunal.

Coercive interventions in law and medicine

Setting the scene

Claire Spivakovsky, Kate Seear and Adrian Carter

The law can have a major impact on an individual's health and wellbeing. The law is the principal tool with which we regulate, contain, empower or advance different populations. One way the law works to produce these effects is through the deployment of targeted coercive medico-legal interventions. Most civil mental health and disability acts, for example, include compulsory treatment and involuntary detention orders. These interventions are used when people with mental illness or disability are adjudged to be at significant risk of harming themselves or others, and are thought to require medical intervention in order to reduce such risk. There are also mandatory alcohol and drug treatment provisions nestled under inebriates acts for 'risky' or 'vulnerable' individuals whose substance use is perceived as causing themselves or others significant harm. And there are specialist jurisdictions under criminal law, such as drug courts or mental health courts, which provide a range of mandated medico-legal interventions for people with mental illness, disability or substance 'addictions' who have fallen foul of the law.

Ostensibly, these examples of what is often termed 'coercive care' seem appropriate, beneficial and benevolent. That is to say, intervening in these populations' lives appears to protect both society and the individuals themselves from experiencing the kinds of harms we have come to associate with certain forms of 'ill-health'. Yet, scholars from a range of disciplines have begun to question these assumptions.

Criminologists and legal scholars, for example, have pointed to the ways that specialist court practices often end up mimicking or becoming even being more intrusive and onerous than traditional forms of punishments (see, for example, Gowan & Whetstone, 2012; Hannah-Moffat & Maurutto, 2012; Moore, 2007). Scholars from psychology, psychiatry and public health have alternatively pointed to the problems with the evidence base underpinning many compulsory forms of treatment in civil law, including the lack of evidence (see, for example, Brophy & McDermott, 2003; Hall, Farrell & Carter, 2014; Kisely & Hall, 2014; Werb et al., 2016). At the same time, human rights scholars have drawn attention to the discriminatory nature of medico-legal interventions, highlighting the incongruence between these targeted forms of coercive treatment and international human rights conventions such as the Convention on the Rights of Persons with Disabilities (see for example, Amon et al., 2013; Callaghan & Ryan, 2016; Nilsson, 2014). In addition, our colleagues from 'mad' and critical disability studies have offered powerful accounts of the significant deleterious effects these interventions have on people's lives, bodies and sense of self (see, for example, Chapman, 2012; Fabris, 2011; Lefrancois, Menzies & Reaume, 2013).

Despite the disquiet that surrounds coercive interventions, they persist. In fact, they are evolving, and in some instances expanding.

Age-old approaches to the coercive containment and control of people with mental illness, disability and/or substance dependence are increasingly being enhanced with new technologies that make these practices more in tune with the modern world. There are, for instance, electronic monitoring devices, such as GPS trackers and alcohol monitoring bracelets, which are now being used to modernise coercive interventions for offenders who have a mental illness or substance dependence (Hearn, 2015; Midgette & Kilmer, 2015). There are also more covert and insidious forms of coercive interventions being introduced into law, with several countries now trialling mandatory drug testing (and coerced abstinence) for welfare recipients, as well as cashless welfare cards that restrict welfare recipients from purchasing alcohol and gambling related products.

Perhaps unsurprisingly, these evolutions in coercive interventions have been met with critique (see Bielefeld, 2012; Dee, 2013; Macdonald et al., 2001), and yet, like their predecessors, they show no signs of abating. For us this raises the question: why do they persist? That is to say, what are the kinds of assumptions, beliefs, logics and evidence bases that sustain the ongoing use and expansion of coercive interventions in contemporary society?

Of course we are not the first to raise these kinds of questions. Several others have interrogated the evidence, logic and appeal of coercive interventions from different perspectives (for a human rights perspective, see McSherry & Freckelton, 2013; for a focus on coercive interventions in community mental health, see Molodynski, Rugkasa & Burns, 2016; for a focus on the coercive nature of drug courts, see Tiger, 2013). However, there is a still a tendency amongst many scholars to write what Mol and Law (2002) would call 'overviews' of coercive interventions: accounts that minimise or shy away from the full complexity and inconvenient multiplicities of these practices. Indeed, there is a tendency amongst scholars to privilege certain kinds of knowledges about coercive interventions over others – with the 'truths' of evidence-based practice often regarded in higher stead than the voices of those subjected to the practice. There is also a tendency to engage with the practice of coercive interventions in a largely siloed fashion, with many scholars focusing on coercive interventions in mental health settings, or coercive interventions in drug and alcohol treatment, but few considering the overlaps, collisions and intersections that occur between these two sectors (a notable exception is Sullivan & O'Donnell, 2012, in the case of post-Independence Ireland). Moreover, there is a habit amongst scholars to preach to the converted, such that it has become rare to hear the voices of those who ultimately support the use of coercive interventions (in some form) alongside and in direct conversation with those who argue for its abolition.

The objective of this edited collection is to hold some of these much-needed conversations about coercive interventions but in a way that does not smooth away or simplify the complexity of the issues involved, nor treat these practices in a narrow fashion. To do this the collection brings together contributions from a range of scholarly disciplines (including criminology, law, ethics, psychology and public health) and combines them with unique accounts from legal and medical practitioners, social-service 'consumers' and government officials. It leaves space for conflicting perspectives on the role and need for coercive interventions to be heard, and it allows for the multiple logics, assumptions and beliefs that surround and operate through these practices to be observed in situ (sometimes disharmoniously).

This is not to suggest, however, that the collection fails to draw connections between diverse practices or ignores overarching themes. Rather, the collection explores the ways in which age-old and contemporary evolutions of coercive interventions intersect with broader, gendered and racialised approaches to governance, offering insights into the unique role coercive medico-legal interventions play in the attempted production of 'good' and 'healthy' citizens. The collection also avoids neat and simplistic conclusions about the phenomena being examined. Instead, the collection seeks to 'sensitise' its readers to the complexities and difficulties associated with these practices. It also aims to inspire writers from other parts of the world to consider whether any of the ideas and insights offered up in this book are translatable to the practices which they encounter. These dual aims are inspired by critical work from the field of science and technology studies, and are ideas that require some explanation.

Critique and complexity

The structure and approach we take in this edited collection is inspired by the work of Annemarie Mol and John Law (2002), including, in particular, their work on 'complexities'. Broadly speaking, Mol and Law's work involves a set of interrelated critiques of research methods and methodologies and academic practice, and seeks to disrupt and destabilise conventional approaches to academic work (of which this collection, of course, is an example). Their starting point is the notion that 'the world is complex' and that 'it escapes simplicities' (p. 1). Crucially, however, they argue that there is a tendency in much academic work to shy away from this complexity, and to instead aspire towards producing 'neat' and 'simplistic' accounts of the world. Mol and Law urge academics to attend to complexity as opposed to seeking to suppress, ignore or overcome it. In other words, they encourage academics to sit with inconsistencies and tensions, with mess and uncertainty, and to treat these phenomena not as 'errors' or 'challenges' to be disregarded, but as proper objects of inquiry and interest. This requires a commitment to doing academic work 'nonreductively, but without at the same time generating ever more complexities until we submerge in chaos' (p. 1). The key insight of their work is: 'That which is complex cannot be pinned down. To pin it down is to lose it' (p. 21).

Of course, this raises the question of how precisely academics work to pin down complexities. How and where do these processes of simplification occur? And how, in an associated sense, might we address them?

A key site for the production of simplification is via the process of *research design*, in which objects and phenomena – among many other things – are typically examined in isolation. In a clinical trial, for instance, forms of treatment for a disease might be tested on a particular population of a certain age and/or gender living with only the specified condition under investigation. In practice, however, the results of such trials may be less useful when dealing with individuals of different ages and genders, or those living with multiple conditions, and for whom the situation is less 'simplistic'.

Another way that simplification is produced is through the *process of academic writing*. Much academic writing utilises the style of 'the overview', in which neat summaries or findings are drawn. The principal problem with overviews is that their production involves deliberate choices – about what to include and what to omit, about what is 'important' or 'significant' and what is not. Importantly, Mol and Law (2002) argue that accounts of this kind are part of the process by which reality is enacted and stabilised. Writing, in this sense, does not *reflect* a pre-existing reality, but instead *constitutes* that reality; a reality that appears to be (and thus *emerges as*) self-contained and ordered. Overviews can create an 'illusion' of order and are thus problematic. This is because a 'single text cannot be everywhere at once. It cannot do everything all at the same time nor tell all' (p. 6).

So where does this leave us? What does it mean if academics should eschew the overview? What are the implications of this for producing an edited collection such as this one which seeks to 'collect' in one place a range of critical perspectives on coercive interventions? Mol and Law (2002) offer up three modes for analysis and writing that steer clear of the simplifying tendencies of conventional academic writing. They call these: 'lists', 'cases' and 'walks'.

The inclusion of lists may seem to be a strange choice, given that conventional lists can sometimes operate as overviews, especially where they 'impose a single mode of ordering' (Mol & Law, 2002, p. 14). In contrast, however, Mol and Law recommend a style that 'abstains from taming', 'remains open' and does not purport to (nor attempt to be) complete. The kind of lists they envisage present information non-hierarchically, without closure, and are open to change.

Cases, on the other hand, are objects of analysis that do not purport to be 'representative of something larger – into which they neatly fit' (Mol & Law, 2002, p. 15). A case may be 'instructive beyond its specific site and situation' but 'what is similar and different [as between sites] is not to be taken for granted' (p. 15). Cases can be used to 'sensitize' readers to events and situations, and may offer potentially 'translatable' insights. They should work as an 'incitement to ask questions about difference and similarity, about what alters in moving from one place to another' (p. 16).

The final option is to utilise the style of 'walks', inspired by the work of Michel de Certeau. The walk is best understood through setting it alongside its counterpart: the map. Maps are a form of overview, insofar as they 'draw surfaces that contain details (a set of sites or attributes of what is contained within these sites) that are related in an accountable manner' (Mol & Law, 2002, p. 16). In contrast, for de Certeau, walking 'is a mode of covering space that gives no overview' – as when one wanders through the little laneways of Venice, or weaves their way through a jungle. Mol and Law (2002) explain:

> As we walk, we may encounter a variety of comforting – or stunning – sights and situations, and then we can bring these together instead or leave them separate, as they would be on a map, removed from one another. We may juxtapose them in the way we sometimes do after a journey, by telling stories or showing pictures. The picture of a large landscape is printed so that it has the same size as that of a plate filled with food, and the story about driving through the landscape is no bigger or smaller than the story about eating the meal. Other differences abound.
>
> (p. 16)

The goal of such an approach is 'to walk and tell stories about this rather than to seek to make maps' (Mol & Law, 2002, p. 17).

We see this edited collection as an exercise in taking walks and telling stories about coercive interventions. In keeping with Mol and Law's concerns about complexity and simplification, this collection invites its audience to take a walk through the terrain of coercive interventions, but not so as to produce a map, or to constitute a view 'from above'. Readers are free to read all or only some of the four parts of the book and, within those parts, all or only some chapters. Readers may also move between chapters in different parts. In this sense, the style and layout of the book are designed to permit (and indeed encourage) walks, whereby readers can wander down little laneways, take turns that interest them, drawing some things together or leaving them separate, as they please. Readers might also tell stories or take pictures of what they observe along the way, but these imprints of knowledge are of the same size; neither is privileged over the other, nor bigger or smaller than another. We argue that this approach not only makes sense given the complex nature of the diverse range of phenomena being studied, but that it represents an important political and ethical intervention into the discourse of coercive interventions. We say this because the collection encourages readers to attend to all forms of articulation, including personal experiences and evidence from clinical trials, in ways that privilege neither.

At the same time, this edited collection also approaches coercive interventions – following Mol and Law's encouragement – as a 'case', or perhaps, more accurately, as a set of *cases*: ones that may have *lessons* for coercive interventions underway in other parts of the world, but without making any claims to *representativeness*. In the instance of this collection, all contributions focus on examples from Australian law and practice. We see this approach as offering two main benefits:

- it releases contributors from the need to devote (and lose) a significant component of their chapter to both outlining the location-specific socio-legal history of their country, and speaking to the influence of this history (or lack thereof) of forms of coercive interventions in law and medicine; and
- it enables the collection as a whole to sensitise readers to an understudied and somewhat neglected set of practices/phenomena: the coexisting and/or divergent logics, assumptions and beliefs that are used to sustain and support the use of coercive interventions within and amongst a range of different populations, including people living with mental illness, disability and/or substance dependence, as well as welfare recipients and children and young people with medical conditions.

Of course, in taking this 'case' approach, and in selecting Australia as the location for examining these practices, we recognise that Australia has its own socio-legal history that influences both the kinds of coercive interventions that are used within this country's borders, and the orientation of these practices. Indeed, while this collection will show how the coercive interventions used in Australia draw upon the same international 'evidence base' that is used around the world and, as such, are consistent with those practices that have taken shape in the USA, UK and most of Europe, it will also illustrate how Australia has its own history of colonisation, its own timeline for women's emancipation and its own penchant for neoliberal welfare reform that shape the practices and purpose of coercion in Australian law and medicine. As such, this collection ultimately invites reflection on how Australian practices may mirror or diverge from those in other parts of the world, and offers its readers potentially translatable ideas and insights for use in their own countries, while still encouraging examinations elsewhere. In Mol and Law's terms, that is, we view this collection as an 'incitement to ask questions about difference and similarity, about what alters in moving from one place to another' (2002, p. 16).

Walking through the collection

For the reasons we have outlined, then, we encourage our readers to approach this collection through the metaphor of 'the walk'. Importantly, Mol and Law (2002) suggest that the process of walking can be aided by techniques of *guidance*:

> a local inhabitant who knows the place and can give directions is much better, and so are signposts that point in the right direction. In the jungle you might need something else to make your path a little simpler: a guide, for sure, but also a sharp machete and the skill to use it.
>
> (p. 16)

To this end, the edited collection is divided into four parts, each preceded by a mini introduction. These are intended to operate as 'signposts' which give a sense of what lies ahead, seek to provoke new ideas and insights, and to guide the readers through the walk they are taking. Like the metaphorical 'machete' in Mol and Law's writing, they are intended to provide our audience with the skills to make the path a little simpler, but without simplifying the issues at hand.

Part I reviews the evidence often used to assess whether coercive treatments are useful, ethical and/or appropriate responses to people with severe mental illnesses, disability or drug addictions. It considers what evidence exists in relation to the effectiveness of coercive interventions in law and medicine, the strengths and limitations of this evidence base, and the reasons why some coercive interventions persist when their foundations are uncertain. Contributors to this part of the book include both academics and medical practitioners, and while each takes a somewhat different stance on the ongoing necessity for coercive interventions, all recognise and call for the need for better evidence and evaluation of coerced treatment programs, and a move away from the current situation which sees coerced treatment policies implemented in response to public concern, political expediency or well-meaning assumptions about their impact on the people treated under various coerced treatment orders.

Of course, questions around the use of coercion in the mental health, disability and alcohol or other drug (AOD) sectors are not simply empirical ones, which is why Part II approaches the issue from a different angle. Focussing on the lives, bodies and voices of those most closely affected by coercive interventions, the chapters in Part II explore the material impacts and lived effects of coercion. Here we hear from a lawyer, mental health 'consumer' and academic who encourage us to confront some uncomfortable questions about coercive treatment and the power of the law. Together, the contributors to this part of the book raise profound and disturbing questions about how we treat some of society's most vulnerable citizens and the harms that might be perpetrated upon them in the names of 'justice' and 'treatment'.

They encourage us to consider: if coercive treatment is inherently unjust, can it ever be warranted?

Unable to draw an uncontested response to this question, Part III continues this collection's walk through critical perspectives on coercive interventions by shifting our attention outward. Specifically it considers how the rationales underpinning decisions to coercively intervene in the lives of certain populations (and not others) might also intersect with overarching and longstanding goals of governance and population management. With contributions from lawyers and academics, the chapters in this third part offer insight into the ways that social processes for producing 'good', 'healthy' and 'productive' lives are not evenly calibrated amongst citizens, and how contemporary medico-legal concerns about bodily control can disguise, deflect and neutralise much older and longstanding processes of population management embedded in law. This observation leaves us with one final question: how might we move forward from here? This is the focus in the final part of the book.

Part IV explores and critiques some of the common paternalistic and protectionist logics which sustain the use of coercive interventions in law and medicine (often in the absence of a strong evidence base). Focusing on specific coercive interventions which are applied to people with mental illness, cognitive impairments and/or AOD addictions, the final part of the book draws out the unexpected and deeply problematic effects that are associated with protecting 'risky' and 'vulnerable' populations from causing harm to themselves or others, and attempts to offer viable alternatives. While each of the contributors in the final part of this collection offer suggestions for reform and reconfiguration, the diversity of the offerings they make ultimately remind us that there is no single way forward from here, and that there is significant scope for other ideas about the evolution or abolition of coercive interventions to be added to this mix.

References

Amon, J., Pearshouse, R., Cohen, J., & Schleifer, R. (2013). Compulsory drug detention centers in China, Cambodia, Vietnam, and Laos: Health and human rights abuses. *Health and Human Rights* 15(2), 124–137.

Bielefeld, S. (2012). Compulsory income management and Indigenous Australians: Delivering social justice or furthering colonial domination? *University of New South Wales Law Journal* 35(2), 522–562.

Brophy, L., & McDermott, F. (2003). What's driving involuntary treatment in the community? The social, policy, legal and ethical context. *Australasian Psychiatry* 11(1), 84–88

Callaghan, S., & Ryan, C. (2016). An evolving revolution: Evaluating Australia's compliance with the Convention on the Rights of Persons with Disabilities in Mental Health Law. *University of New South Wales Law Journal* 39(2), 596–624.

Chapman, C. (2012). Colonialism, disability, and possible lives: The residential treatment of children whose parents survived Indian Residential Schools. *Journal of Progressive Human Services* 23(2), 127–158.

Dee, M. (2013). Welfare surveillance, income management and new paternalism in Australia. *Surveillance & Society* 11(3), 272–286.

Fabris, E. (2011). *Tranquil prisons: Chemical incarceration under community treatment orders.* Toronto: University of Toronto Press.

Gowan, T., & Whetstone, S. (2012). Making the criminal addict: Subjectivity and social control in a strong-arm rehab. *Punishment & Society* 14(1), 69–93.

Hall, W., Farrell, M. & Carter, A., (2014). Compulsory treatment of addiction in the patient's best interests: More rigorous evaluations are essential. *Drug and Alcohol Review* 33(3), 268–271.

Hannah-Moffat, K., & Maurutto, P. (2012). Shifting and targeted forms of penal governance: Bail, punishment and specialized courts. *Theoretical Criminology* 16(2), 201–219.

Hearn, D. (2015). Other GPS uses: Forensic mental health. *Probation Quarterly, Issue 5, Electronic Monitoring.* http://probation-institute.org/other-gps-uses-forensic-mental-health/ (accessed 16 October 2017).

Kisely, S., & Hall, K. (2014). An updated meta-analysis of randomized controlled evidence for the effectiveness of community treatment orders. *The Canadian Journal of Psychiatry* 59(10), 561–564.

Lefrancois, B., Menzies, R., & Reaume, G. (2013). *Mad matters: A critical reader in Canadian mad studies.* Toronto: Canadian Scholars' Press Inc.

Macdonald, S., Bois, C., Brands, B., Dempsey, D., Erickson, P., Marsh, D., Meredith, S., Shain, M., Skinner, W., & Chiu, A. (2001). Drug testing and mandatory treatment for welfare recipients. *International Journal of Drug Policy* 12(3), 249–257.

McSherry, B., & Freckelton, I. (Eds.) (2013). *Coercive care: Rights, law and policy.* London: Routledge.

Midgette, G., & Kilmer, B. (2015). *The effect of Montana's 24/7 sobriety program on DUI Re-arrest: Insights from a natural experiment with limited administrative data.* Santa Monica, CA: RAND Corporation. www.rand.org/pubs/working_papers/WR1083.html (accessed 23 January 2017).

Molodynski, A., Rugkasa, J., & Burns, T. (Eds.) (2016). *Coercion in community mental health care: International perspectives.* Oxford: Oxford University Press.

Mol, A., & Law, J. (2002). Complexities: An introduction. In J. Law & A. Mol (Eds.), *Complexities: Social studies of knowledge practices* (pp. 1–22). Durham, NC: Duke University Press.

Moore, D. (2007). Translating justice and therapy: The Drug Treatment Court networks. *British Journal of Criminology* 47(1), 42–60.

Nilsson, A. (2014). Objective and reasonable? Scrutinising compulsory mental health interventions from a non-discrimination perspective. *Human Rights Law Review* 14(3), 459–485.

Sullivan, E., & O'Donnell, I. (2012). *Coercive confinement in Ireland: Patients, prisoners and penitents.* Manchester: Manchester University Press.

Tiger, R. (2013). *Judging addicts: Drug courts and coercion in the justice system.* New York, NY: New York University Press.

Werb, D., Kamarulzaman, A., Meacham, M., Rafful, B., Fischer, B., Strathdee, S., & Wood, E. (2016). The effectiveness of compulsory drug treatment: A systematic review. *International Journal of Drug Policy* 28, 1–9.

Part I

Examining foundations for coercive interventions in law and medicine

Part I of this book reviews the evidence often used to assess whether coercive treatments are useful, ethical or appropriate responses to people with severe mental illnesses, disability or drug addictions. As we will see in subsequent chapters of the book, questions around the use of coercion in the mental health, disability and alcohol or other drug (AOD) sectors are not simply empirical ones, but need to examine a constellation of moral, social and legal issues. However, an initial requirement for the use of any form of coerced treatment is evidence that it is effective in benefiting the person who is being coerced. The use of coerced 'treatment' without evidence of its safety and effectiveness could amount to some form of extrajudicial punishment or harmful discrimination of vulnerable persons. Part I examines the evidence base underpinning the use of coercive medico-legal interventions in mental health and AOD addictions around the world. It considers what evidence exists in relation to the effectiveness of coercive interventions in law and medicine, the strengths and limitations of this evidence base, and the reasons why some coercive interventions persist when their foundations are uncertain. Notably absent from this part of the book is a chapter about the evidence base for coercive interventions in the disability sector and the questions it raises. This absence is not an oversight nor an omission, but rather a reflection on the current state of affairs within this sector.

There is a wide range of evidence that can and is deployed in support, or critique, of coerced forms of medical interventions. The first two chapters of Part I of the book consider key empirical questions regarding the use of coercion in mental health care: first, is the person experiencing a condition that justifies the use of coercion, and second, is the form of coerced treatment being provided effective in improving the wellbeing of the person being coerced into treatment?

The decision-making capacity of people with severe mental illness or drug addictions is often central to debates about the appropriate use of coercion in mental health care. Support for coercive interventions often relies on paternalistic justifications that those with some mental illnesses are unable to make appropriate decisions regarding their health and well-being, and should therefore be treated for their own good. In Chapter 1, Carter and Hall examine evidence that people with drug addictions are so cognitively impaired by their addiction that they are unable to make autonomous decisions about drug use and its treatment. Proponents of coerced addiction treatment increasingly rely on insights from neuroscience research to suggest that the brains of people who are severely addicted to drugs have been 'hijacked' by that drug and need to be coerced into treatment for their own good. Carter and Hall examine the evidence in support of this claim, arguing that it is incorrect and misleading to argue that people with addictions have no control over their drug use.

In Chapter 2, Brophy, Ryan and Weller carefully examine whether coerced treatment of people with mental illness is effective. They specifically examine whether the use of community treatment orders (CTOs), also known as assisted outpatient treatment, is effective in improving the health and well-being of people with mental illness. These treatment orders came into favour following the demise of large psychiatric institutions and community concerns about relapse and revolving door admissions. Despite their widespread use in many parts of the globe, Brophy and colleagues demonstrate that there is very little evidence that these programs are effective. What limited evidence is available does not employ robust methods or adequate follow-ups to answer the question of whether CTOs actually work. They then consider another form of evidence relevant to debates about whether coerced treatment is ethical: the lived experiences of those who are subject to them. These themes are explored in greater detail in Part II.

In the concluding chapter of Part I, Batey provides another kind of evidence. Batey is a drug and alcohol clinician, and he writes his chapter from the perspective of a drug and alcohol clinician desperately trying to save the lives of his patients who are acutely threatened by their continued use of alcohol. In Chapter 3, Batey describes several clear examples of the immediate threats to a person's health and wellbeing that compulsory alcohol treatment seeks to address. These case studies provide a compelling picture of the good that coerced treatment orders aim to achieve, when they are operated by sympathetic individuals whose primary motivation is the health and wellbeing of their patient.

A common theme running throughout these chapters is the considerable lack of adequate evidence with which to assess the effectiveness of coerced treatment. Studies are poorly designed, with insufficient follow-up of participants. Often policies are widely employed on the basis of little evidence. While the authors of these chapters may interpret this lack of adequate evidence differently, they all recognise and call for the need for better evidence and evaluation of coerced treatment programs, and a move away from the current situation which sees coerced treatment policies implemented in response to public concern, political expediency or well-meaning assumptions about their impact on the people treated under various coerced treatment orders. Conflicting aims of coerced treatment to both assist and treat unwell individuals and protect society from real or perceived harms can undermine both the type and quality of treatment that people receive. All of the authors provide a clear way forward for obtaining the necessary evidence for establishing whether coerced treatment is ethical, whether it works and how it may be done in a way that maximises both.

Chapter 1

From coerced to compulsory treatment of addiction in the patient's best interests

Is it supported by the evidence?

Adrian Carter and Wayne Hall

There is good evidence that those who enter treatment for drug addictions[1] or problematic drug use will benefit from the treatment (Gerstein & Harwood, 1990). However, a persistent problem in treating addiction is attracting people with serious drug use disorders into treatment and keeping them there long enough for them to benefit from the encounter (see Chapter 3, this volume). The reluctance of many drug-dependent persons to enter treatment has led governments at various times to legally coerce people with addictions into treatment by offering it as an alternative to imprisonment for those who have committed criminal offences. Proponents of this approach argue that coerced addiction treatment is justified because it reduces the harm to people with addictions and the harmful effects of their addiction on their families and friends, and their social and economic impacts on society (Chandler et al., 2009; Sullivan et al., 2008). Others have argued for the use of compulsory treatment rather than coercion into treatment, asserting that individuals with serious forms of addiction are so overwhelmed by their condition that the community is morally obliged to compel them to enter addiction treatment for their own good (Caplan, 2008).

Critics of coerced treatment oppose it for various reasons. For some it is unethical because they believe that people who use drugs make free and fully informed choices to use drugs and should not be prevented from doing so. If drug users commit criminal offences, they should be treated in the same way as other offenders (Foddy & Savulescu, 2006a; Szasz, 1975). Some argue that coerced treatment does not work or can cause more harm than benefit (Wild, 2006).

In this chapter we address the following questions: can legal coercion be used ethically and effectively to treat drug addiction? If so, under what conditions is it ethical to do so? We begin by briefly reviewing the various ways in which coercion or compulsion may be used, and examine the ethical arguments offered in favour of the use of coerced treatment. We examine the plausibility of neurobiological explanations of addiction that have been used in recent years to justify forced addiction treatment. We then suggest some guidelines for the ethical use of coercion in the treatment of addiction, including compulsory treatment.

A taxonomy of coerced addiction treatment

A distinction is often drawn between voluntary (freely chosen) and involuntary (compelled) treatment of addiction. In reality, addicted persons rarely decide to enter treatment entirely freely. Internal forces (such as withdrawal symptoms) and external pressures from family and friends or workmates may prompt a decision to seek treatment. Coerced addiction treatment may vary in the amount of force used to encourage treatment entry and, therefore, the degree to which an individual's liberty, freedom and autonomy is affected.[2]

Informal mild coercion includes social pressure from friends and family to enter treatment (Maddux, 1988). Social coercion can be an effective motivation to enter treatment (Wild et al., 1998). Addiction can place an enormous emotional and financial burden on families and friends so it is not surprising that loved ones motivate treatment seeking by highlighting the destructive impact of the person's behaviour on the family. People with problematic drug use may not fully appreciate the impact that they are having on themselves or others. Social pressure from family and friends to cease drug use often provides the first external indication that drug use is problematic.

Unfortunately, for some people with long-term drug problems, important social ties have often been severed or no longer influence their lives. More formal types of coercion that do not involve the criminal justice system may come from employers who make it a condition of continued employment that an employee with a substance use disorder undergoes treatment. Formal non-criminal coercion by employers and other nongovernmental agencies, such as Employment Assistance Programs in the US, are negotiated between agencies or employers and the individual. The ethical guidelines for how these programs operate are codified in the appropriate laws (e.g., industrial relations, professional codes of conduct). Physicians may be required to undergo treatment for an addiction in order to retain their license to practice (McLellan et al., 2008).

While informal social coercion and formal non-criminal coercion represent very important drivers for entering treatment, they arguably raise fewer ethical issues in the treatment of dependence than legally mandated treatment. In both cases, the dependent person can either agree to treatment or suffer the threatened consequences, such as the loss of employment or relationship. The form of coercion that raises the ethical concerns that will be the topic for the remainder of this chapter is legal coercion, in which a person is either encouraged to enter treatment under the threat of imprisonment, or legal force is used to mandate the treatment of their addiction (Klag et al., 2005).

The form of legal coercion that has become increasingly popular within the criminal justice system is the use of diversionary programs that offer drug addicted offenders treatment as an alternative to imprisonment. This can occur at various stages in the criminal justice process (Pritchard et al., 2007). In the first instance, treatment may be offered before being charged by police; this is not an ideal method of coercion, because it falls outside judicial oversight. It is possible that relying on the discretion of police opens the way to individuals being coerced into treatment for reasons other than criminal behaviour, such as behaving in an unconventional way or being a member of a social minority (Hall, 1997).

Legally coerced treatment is most often advocated for persons either charged with, or convicted of, an offence to which their drug dependence has contributed. It is generally offered as an alternative to imprisonment in order to have legal sanctions deferred, reduced or lifted, or as a condition of parole (Klag et al., 2005; Rotgers, 1992). Suspension of legal sanctions is usually made conditional upon successful completion of a treatment program, with the penalty of imprisonment if the person fails to comply (Hall, 1997). Each of these forms of legally coerced treatment have different legal and social consequences for the offenders subjected to them, and they require varying degrees of deprivation of liberty, restraint and hardship.

The ethics of legally coerced treatment

A major justification for legally coerced addiction treatment is that treating addicted offenders will reduce the likelihood of reoffending (Chandler et al., 2009). The strongest evidence comes from the treatment of opioid dependence, where studies have shown that treatment of heroin addiction significantly reduces criminal behaviour while participants remain in treatment (Gerstein & Harwood, 1990). Similar (although less compelling) results are seen in people treated for alcohol and amphetamine dependence (Chandler et al., 2009). The use of drug treatment programs as an alternative to incarceration has also been motivated by the failure of prison terms to reduce drug use and drug-related crime, and by the over-representation of drug-dependent people in prisons (Hall, 1997).

The advent of HIV/AIDS provided an additional argument for treating drug addiction (Dolan et al., 1996). Keeping people who inject drugs out of prison reduces the transmission of infectious diseases such as HIV and the hepatitis C virus (HCV) while in detention and following release from prison. People who inject drugs in prison are at significantly increased risk of contracting bloodborne viruses – and potentially spreading the viruses to the wider population upon release – because of a lack of access to sterile injecting equipment in most prisons (Small et al., 2005; Wood et al., 2005). The incidence of HIV and HCV is also significantly higher in prison populations than the wider public (Dolan et al., 2006). The ethical, correctional and public health arguments for drug treatment under coercion are reinforced by the economic argument that it is less costly to treat drug-dependent offenders in the community than to imprison them (Gerstein & Harwood, 1990).

The public health and personal benefits of coerced treatment, however, are not sufficient to justify its use. Coerced treatment overrides an individual's autonomous decision-making and this requires a strong ethical justification. Coerced treatment of addiction is often justified on the grounds that people with a drug addiction are unable to make a free decision about their drug use, by virtue of being addicted, and hence may be coerced into treatment because it is in their best interests, or for their 'own good'. The use of paternalistically coerced treatment could be seen as justified if addicted individuals suffered from a condition that robbed them of their autonomy and impaired their capacity to choose not to use drugs. Developments in neuroscience research of addiction have been used to provide a neurobiological rationale for this view (Caplan, 2008; Charland, 2002; Cohen, 2002). We examine the impact of addiction on an individual's autonomy below.

Two models of addiction

A central question in debates about the coerced or mandated treatment of addiction is whether addicted individuals have the capacity to make free choices about their drug use. We review two contrasting views that have dominated recent public debates about this issue: the medical model, in which addiction is seen as 'a chronic relapsing brain disease' that hijacks a person's capacity to control their drug use (Dackis & O'Brien, 2005); and the common-sense moral view, which is sceptical about the idea of addiction and sees both drug use, and any criminal acts engaged in to support it, as freely chosen acts for which offenders should be held morally and legally responsible (Szasz, 1975).[3]

The brain disease model of addiction

Advocates of the brain disease model of addiction argue that chronic drug use significantly impairs an individual's ability to control their drug use (Volkow et al., 2016). People with a drug addiction are, in this view, 'hijacked' by their drug (Dackis & O'Brien, 2005). Several bodies of empirical evidence are cited in support of this view.

First, a significant minority of people who use drugs become addicted to them, and the size of this minority depends on the drug, the way in which it is used (e.g., whether swallowed, smoked or injected) and its pharmacological actions (e.g., whether its effects have a fast or slow onset and offset) (Anthony & Helzer, 1991). Generally, drugs that are injected or smoked, that act quickly and for a short period of time (e.g., heroin, cocaine and nicotine), are more likely to produce addictive behaviour than drugs that have a slower onset, act for longer and are taken orally (e.g., codeine, methylphenidate).

Second, it is possible to identify individuals who are more likely to develop an addiction if they use drugs. Twin and adoption studies suggest that genetic factors make a substantial contribution to addiction liability (Ball, 2008). Genetic factors have been estimated to account for between 40% and 60% of addiction liability (Uhl et al., 2008).

Third, neuroimaging studies suggest that the brains of addicted and non-addicted persons differ in how they respond to drugs and drug-related stimuli (Volkow et al., 2014). Addicted individuals also perform worse on neurocognitive tests of decision-making in ways that are correlated with the amount of drugs that have been used and with self-reported cravings for drugs (Baler & Volkow, 2006). These changes often persist for months after abstinence has been achieved, and they are thought to be mediated by increased dopamine activity in the brain's reward pathway (Volkow et al., 2016).

Neuroimaging studies provide a bridge between animal models of addiction and the addictive behaviour of humans. The neurobiological view that addiction arises from repeated effects of drugs on the brain's dopaminergic reward pathway has recently been supported by reports of addictive disorders arising from therapeutic use of dopaminergic drugs in Parkinson's disease (Ambermoon et al., 2011).

Leading addiction clinicians argue that neuroscience research challenges the assumption that addictive behaviour is a voluntary choice (Baler & Volkow, 2006; Dackis & O'Brien, 2005). Prolonged drug use, they argue, produces changes in brain function that persist after abstinence and undermine the capacity of people with an addiction to control their drug use. On this view, people with an addiction lack the autonomous decision-making capacity to choose not to use their drug of addiction, and may need to be forced into treatment to reinstate their autonomy (Caplan, 2008).

The choice model of addiction

The choice or moral model is sceptical about the reality of addiction and sees persons with addictions as people who knowingly and willingly choose to use drugs. Addiction is often seen as an excuse to evade responsibility for socially deviant behaviour that harms others (Satel & Lilienfeld, 2014; Szasz, 1975).

The choice view of drug use makes sense of several features of the behaviour of drug-using offenders. Drug use is, at least initially, a choice and drug users often engage in considerable planning to obtain their drugs (Foddy & Savulescu, 2006b). The fact that addictive patterns of drug use occur in a minority of drug users is explained by the characteristics of these drug users and the environments in which they live rather than by the effects of the drugs that they use (Heyman, 2009). These theorists argue that most people who become dependent on drugs stop without professional assistance (Heyman, 2009). Even severely addicted individuals will cease using drugs if offered small incentives for doing so (e.g., shopping vouchers or cash for drug free urine samples) (Marteau et al., 2009; Petry et al., 2011). Their drug use also responds to lifestyle changes (Heyman, 2009) and changes in drug availability and price (Room, 2007).

How plausible is the brain disease model of addiction?

The primary evidence for a brain disease model of addiction comes from laboratory animal models. Typically animals are trained to self-administer addictive drugs at a high rate, and this behaviour can be shown to resist extinction after the drug is withdrawn. These animal models have good face validity, but their relevance to human compulsive drug use and the contexts in which humans typically use addictive drugs has been questioned (Ahmed, 2010; Ahmed, 2012). Getting rodents 'hooked' on drugs is surprisingly difficult unless the animals are selectively bred to be more easily addicted. Moreover, many of these addictive behaviours (e.g., self-administration, conditioned-place preference, cue-induced reinstatement) disappear when animals are placed in more natural environments for the species, such as those that include littermates and access to a range of alternative activities such as running wheels (Ahmed, 2010; Ahmed, 2012; Alexander et al., 1981).

Neuroimaging and neurocognitive studies of addiction in humans also have major limitations. First, these findings only reflect average group differences between addicted and non-addicted populations. It is not clear that the observed changes in brain and cognition undermine autonomous decision-making in addicted individuals. These studies find that addicted individuals, as a group, have diminished neurocognitive capacity compared with non-addicted individuals, but not all people with an addiction show these deficits, while some non-addicted persons do (Bechara, 2005). Second, these studies are typically cross-sectional, so it is not clear whether the observed changes in brain function are causes or consequences of addictive drug use or some combination of the two (Schumann, 2007).

The claim that addictive drug use is compulsive is inconsistent with behavioural evidence that even people with severe drug use problems retain some degree of control over their drug use (Heyman, 2009). This includes the types of evidence outlined previously, namely, that many, if not most, addicted individuals in the general population overcome their addiction without treatment (Heyman, 2009), and that many addicted persons cease using drugs without assistance for varying periods (e.g., to reduce their tolerance, to take time out from a drug-using lifestyle) or in response to major life events (e.g., the birth of a child, ultimatums from friends and family, or threats from employers) (Heyman, 2009). The fact that small incentives such as vouchers can reduce drug use in addicted persons is especially difficult to reconcile with the claim that a person's drug use is the result of compulsions that are impossible to resist.

When would coerced treatment of addiction be ethical?

Can we reconcile these conflicting perspectives on problem drug use? We agree that people with drug use disorders are not, by definition, unable to make autonomous, rational decisions about whether to use a drug or not. However, we also acknowledge that chronic drug use may affect brain function and cognition in ways that can make decisions not to use drugs more difficult for these persons. The courts in many Western countries (e.g. Australia, the United States, the United Kingdom) often seem to act on a compromise view that reflects this position. Convicted offenders with a drug addiction are often offered treatment as an alternative to punishment for the crimes for which they have been convicted. The suspension or reduction of sentences for crimes that would otherwise receive custodial sentences signals the courts' recognition that addiction can impair offenders' decision-making in ways that may make them less deserving of custodial sentences than other persons who commit the same offences. It also allows society to benefit from the reduced recidivism and better public health consequences that legally coerced treatment allows.

Some commentators have questioned the effectiveness of coerced drug treatment (Gostin, 1993; Newman, 1974; Wild, 1999). Treatment under coercion would be unethical if it were ineffective. Even if treatment under coercion is effective, it may not mean that it should be provided; for example, the community might place a higher value on punishing than rehabilitating offenders (Hall, 1997).

We support the consensus view on drug treatment under legal coercion prepared for the World Health Organization (WHO) (Porter et al., 1986). This argues that legally coerced treatment is ethically justified if and only if: (1) the rights of the individuals are protected by due process (in accordance with human rights principles); and (2) effective and humane treatment is provided. Due process would require some form of judicial oversight of the coerced treatment process. In the absence of due process, coerced treatment could easily become de facto imprisonment without judicial oversight. In the absence of humane care and effectiveness, coerced 'drug treatment' would not meet the WHO ethico-legal standard, and could become a cost-cutting exercise (given that it is less expensive to coercively treat than to imprison people with an addiction who are convicted of offences).

What might an ethical legally coerced treatment program look like?

The uncertain benefits of coerced treatment have led some proponents to argue that offenders should be allowed two 'constrained choices' (Fox, 1992).[4] The first constrained choice for an offender would be whether to participate in drug treatment. If they decline to be treated, they would be dealt with by the criminal justice system in the same way as anyone else charged with their offence. Those who agreed to be treated would be offered a second constrained choice of the type of addiction treatment. There is some empirical support for these recommendations, in that coerced treatment that requires some degree of voluntary interest on the part of the offender appears to be more effective than treatment without any choice (Gerstein & Harwood, 1990).

The constrained choice condition has three implications. First, pharmacological treatment options, including agonist maintenance, should be included in the options offered to coerced individuals. There has been a tendency for coerced treatment programs, particularly in the US, to only offer abstinence-oriented treatment. The manufacturer of Vivitrol, a long-acting opioid antagonist, has recently successfully marketed this product to the US criminal justice system to increase its use in custodial settings (Walsh, 2017). This policy prevents opioid-addicted offenders from accessing the forms of treatment that are most likely to benefit them, such as methadone or buprenorphine maintenance (Hall, 1997; Hall & Lucke, 2010). Second, there should be a range of drug-free treatment options available for those who do not wish to use pharmacological treatment. Third, the safety, effectiveness and cost-effectiveness of whatever forms of treatment that are offered should be rigorously evaluated (National Research Council, 2001).

Ethical issues in coerced addiction treatment also arise from the interaction between the correctional and drug treatment systems (Rotgers, 1992; Skene, 1987). A major problem is the conflict between the expectations of correctional and treatment personnel about the effectiveness of drug treatment and each other's roles and responsibilities. Treatment staff usually regard the drug offender as a client, that is, someone who should be involved in treatment decisions and whose personal information should be respected. Treatment staff also anticipate that their clients will relapse to drug use, and understand that such relapses should be dealt with therapeutically rather than punitively. Correctional and judicial personnel, by contrast, often expect treatment to produce enduring abstinence. They see treatment as under the control of the court, and hence regard any drug use in treatment as an offence that treatment staff are legally obliged to report to the court. When these very different expectations of treatment effectiveness are not met, and there is little communication between courts and treatment services, judges and magistrates may become sceptical about the value of coerced treatment and reduce their use of it (Skene, 1987). Accordingly, the effective and ethical use of coerced drug treatment requires a shared understanding of the likely benefits of treatment and a clear statement of the roles of correctional and treatment staff. The latter should include agreement upon their respective responsibilities for monitoring and reporting upon an offender's progress in drug treatment. Ideally, these issues should be addressed in written protocols that govern interactions between courts and treatment personnel.

Compulsory treatment of addiction

Paternalistically motivated compulsory treatment occurs when addicted individuals who have not committed any offence (apart from being repeatedly intoxicated in public) are compelled to enter treatment, usually by order of a court or a quasi-judicial body, for their own good or the good of family members. Compulsory addiction treatment generally involves the confinement of individuals in specialised drug-treatment facilities, or prison hospitals, usually with the goal of attaining abstinence from drugs (see Chapter 3, this volume). Upon successful completion of an abstinence program, individuals may be released from the facility into some sort of intensely supervised outpatient facility. Failure to comply with any condition of the program usually results in being readmitted to a secure inpatient facility (Gostin, 1993).

For over a century, many jurisdictions have permitted persons with severe addiction to be compulsorily treated in this way. Involuntary treatment of inebriety was introduced in Australia and some US states in the mid to late 19th century. It largely fell out of favour in the 20th century because of its high cost and low success rates (Webb, 2003). Switzerland still allows civil commitment of people with an addiction, but these comprised less than 2% of all admissions in the late 1990s (Grichting et al., 2002). Sweden has had a compulsory treatment system for alcohol and drug dependence for over a century, but the number of persons coming under these provisions has declined in the past decade (Palm & Stenius, 2002). Legislation in many US states allows the civil commitment of people with an addiction, but these provisions are rarely used (Gostin, 1993).

There has been renewed advocacy in Australia (DLA Piper Australia, 2014; PwC's Indigenous Consulting with Menzies School of Health Research, 2017) and the US (Chandler et al., 2009) for the revival of compulsory treatment of severely addicted persons for their own good, particularly in response to increased reporting of crimes associated with crystal methamphetamine use (Lee, 2015). The reasons for this revival are unclear but probably include a convergence of factors. These include the frustration that emergency health care providers experience in dealing with repeated hospital presentations for alcohol and drug-related problems, and pressure from families for the health system to intervene to interrupt the self-destructive alcohol and drug use of their members (Dekker, O'Brien, & Smith, 2010).

Because compulsory treatment involves a maximal deprivation of liberty, it requires a strong ethical justification. Arguably this should include strong evidence that this form of treatment is safe and effective and that the consequences of not treating the person are serious and highly likely to occur (Aronowitz, 1967; Childress et al., 2002).

How effective is compulsory addiction treatment?

A major problem shared by all forms of paternalistic coerced addiction treatment is the lack of evidence about its safety and efficacy. There are no randomised controlled trials or well-controlled observational studies showing that persons who have been compulsorily treated have lower rates of re-hospitalisation, premature death and morbidity than addicted persons who have not been compulsorily treated (Broadstock et al., 2008; New South Wales Standing Committee on Social Issues, 2004). The only evidence for the effectiveness of compulsory addiction treatment are small case series of patients who have been treated in this way (Broadstock et al., 2008; New South Wales Standing Committee on Social Issues, 2004). These studies are unable to consider what might have happened if these individuals had not been compulsorily treated, or if they had been encouraged to enter treatment via other means.

Another concern with the use of compulsory treatment is the effect it has on the ability for those seeking treatment to find it. It makes little sense if the provision of treatment places for compulsory treatment reduces the avail-ability of places for those voluntarily seeking it (Hall, 1997; Leukefeld & Tims, 1988). Compulsory treatment programs can also increase the burden on programs that are effective, well funded and well resourced, adversely affect-ing staff morale and hampering effective treatment centres (Hall, 1997). Governments that choose to reintroduce compulsory addiction treatments must rigorously evaluate how these programs operate, including their long-term effects, using rigorous methodological designs (e.g., randomisation and control groups). They also need to examine their impact on voluntary or legally coerced forms of addiction treatment.

Given the evidence presented above, it is hard to justify the use of com-pulsory treatment for either paternalistic or public good reasons (Leukefeld & Tims, 1988). Compulsory treatment programs abolish the autonomy of the individual, and arguably constitute a violation of civil liberties in a manner that contravenes the International Bill of Human Rights (United Nations, 1976). In a recent report, the United Nations Office on Drugs and Crime (UNODC) argued that compulsory treatment of drug addiction without consent was not only ineffective in treating problem drug use, but comprised a form of imprisonment that violated international human rights agreements (UNODC, 2010).

Conclusion

In some circumstances, coercing individuals into treatment can be an ethically acceptable and effective method of helping someone overcome addiction, as well as providing economic and public welfare benefits for society. Such a view was recognised in a recent UNODC discussion paper arguing that legally coerced treatment of addiction, but not compulsory treatment, is an acceptable alternative to imprisonment that is consistent with several international drug control conventions (e.g., the Single Convention on Narcotic Drugs from 1961) and supported by evidence of effectiveness (UNODC, 2010).

Nevertheless, the use of coerced treatment should not be at the expense of an individual's human and civil rights or used to inappropriately deprive persons of their liberty. The most ethically defensible form of coerced treatment is as an alternative to punishment when an addicted person has been convicted of a crime to which their addiction contributed. Treatment may be offered as an alternative to incarceration, with the threat of imprisonment should they fail to comply with the treatment program. Offenders should still have the choice of the form of treatment that they receive, with all forms of effective treatment being made available. Not all individuals respond positively to the same treatment, and offenders are likely to benefit from an approach in which they have a personal investment. This 'choice' serves both ethical and pragmatic purposes.

Coerced treatment should also be seen as an opportunity to engage with addicted individuals who are often socially isolated and to create cohesion between health care systems and addicted persons (UNODC, 2010). These programs should minimise the use of coercive measures and maximise the autonomy of addicted individuals. When coercion is used it should be with the aim of treating a medical condition, by providing a choice of effective treatments, not as a form of extrajudicial punishment. Punitive, coercive policies are not only unethical; they often produce more harm to society and the individual than less coercive treatment approaches.

Notes

1 We use the term 'addiction' in this chapter to describe a pattern of drug use that causes significant harms to a person, and which they are unable to suppress or reduce despite numerous attempts and a strong desire to do so. We acknowledge the complex and socially constructed nature of definitions of various forms of drug use that people describe as 'problematic'. We are unable to examine the contested nature of the terms used to describe problematic drug use in this chapter, and use the terms addiction, dependence and drug or substance use disorders interchangeably. See Chapter 5, this volume.
2 See Chapter 5, this volume.
3 We acknowledge that there is a wider range of views or models of drug use than the two presented here. We have contrasted the medical or disease model and the choice or moral model because they represent two extreme perspectives on drug use that are commonly contrasted and debated in the literature. We acknowledge that neither model provides an accurate or complete account of addictive drug use, but they do provide an important framework for understanding the ethical issues at stake. We also think it is important to thoughtfully critique the accuracy of the brain disease model of addiction which has come to dominate addiction treatment and policy in many countries, particularly the US.

4   There is something of a contradiction in the notion of a 'constrained' choice. Is it really a choice if it is constrained? In reality most choices are constrained to some degree, yet we still refer to them as choices. It could be argued that the notion of a truly free and unconstrained choice is an unrealistic ideal that is not realised in the social and neurobiological world in which choices are taken.

References

Ahmed, S. H. (2010). Validation crisis in animal models of drug addiction: beyond non-disordered drug use toward drug addiction. *Neuroscience & Biobehavioral Reviews* 35, 172–184.

Ahmed, S. H. (2012). The science of making drug-addicted animals. *Neuroscience* 211, 107–125.

Alexander, B. K., Beyerstein, B. L., Hadaway, P. F., & Coambs, R. B. (1981). Effect of early and later colony housing on oral ingestion of morphine in rats. *Pharmacology, Biochemistry and Behavior* 15, 571–576.

Ambermoon, P., Carter, A., Hall, W., Dissanayaka, N. N. W., & O'Sullivan, J. D. (2011). Impulse control disorders in patients with Parkinson's disease receiving dopamine replacement therapy: evidence and implications for the addictions field. *Addiction* 106, 283–293.

Anthony, J. C., & Helzer, J. (1991). Syndromes of drug abuse and dependence. In L. N. Robins & D. A. Regier (Eds.), *Psychiatric disorders in America*. New York: Academic Press.

Aronowitz, D. (1967). Civil commitment of narcotics addicts. *Columbia Law Review* 67, 405–429.

Baler, R. D., & Volkow, N. D. (2006). Drug addiction: the neurobiology of disrupted self-control. *Trends in Molecular Medicine* 12, 559–566.

Ball, D. (2008). Addiction science and its genetics. *Addiction* 103, 360–367.

Bechara, A. (2005). Decision making, impulse control and loss of willpower to resist drugs: a neurocognitive perspective. *Nature Neuroscience*, 8, 1458–1463.

Broadstock, M., Brinson, D., & Weston, A. (2008). *The effectiveness of compulsory, residential treatment of chronic alcohol or drug addiction in non-offenders: a systematic review of the literature*. Canterbury: University of Canterbury, Health Services Assessment Collaboration (HSAC).

Caplan, A. (2008). Denying autonomy in order to create it: the paradox of forcing treatment upon addicts. *Addiction* 103, 1919–1921.

Chandler, R. K., Fletcher, B. W., & Volkow, N. D. (2009). Treating drug abuse and addiction in the criminal justice system: improving public health and safety. *JAMA* 301, 183–190.

Charland, L. C. (2002). Cynthia's dilemma: consenting to heroin prescription. *American Journal of Bioethics* 2, 37–47.

Childress, J. F., Faden, R. R., Gaare, R. D., Gostin, L. O., Kahn, J., Bonnie, R. J., Kass, N. E., Mastroianni, A. C., Moreno, J. D., & Nieburg, P. (2002). Public health ethics: mapping the terrain. *Journal of Law Medicine & Ethics* 30, 170–178.

Cohen, P. J. (2002). Untreated addiction imposes an ethical bar to recruiting addicts for non-therapeutic studies of addictive drugs. *Journal of Law Medicine & Ethics* 30, 73–81.

Dackis, C., & O'Brien, C. (2005). Neurobiology of addiction: treatment and public policy ramifications. *Nature Neuroscience* 8, 1431–1436.

Dekker, J., O'Brien, K., & Smith, N. (2010). *An evaluation of the Compulsory Drug Treatment Program (CDTP)*. Sydney: NSW Bureau of Crime Statistics and Research.

DLA Piper Australia (2014). *Review of the Severe Substance Dependence Treatment Act 2014 (Vic): Volume 1*. Melbourne: Victorian Department of Health.

Dolan, K., Kite, B., Black, E., Aceijas, C., & Stimson, G. V. (2006). HIV in prison in low-income and middle-income countries. *The Lancet Infectious Diseases* 7, 32–41.

Dolan, K., Wodak, A., Hall, W., Gaughin, M., & Rae, F. (1996). HIV risk behaviour of injecting drug users before, during and after imprisonment in New South Wales. *Addictive Research* 4, 151–160.

Foddy, B., & Savulescu, J. (2006a). *Addiction* and autonomy: can addicted people consent to the prescription of their drug of addiction? *Bioethics* 20, 1–15.

Foddy, B., & Savulescu, J. (2006b). Autonomy, addiction and the drive to pleasure: designing drugs and our biology: a reply to Neil Levy. *Bioethics* 20, 21–23.

Fox, R. G. (1992). The compulsion of voluntary treatment in sentencing. *Criminal Law Journal* 16, 37–54.

Gerstein, D. R., & Harwood, H. J. (1990). *Treating drug problems (Volume 1). A study of effectiveness and financing of public and private drug treatment systems*. Washington, DC: Institute of Medicine, National Academy Press.

Gostin, L. O. (1993). Compulsory treatment for drug-dependent persons: justifications for a public health approach to drug dependency. In R. Bayer & G. M. Oppenheimer (Eds.), *Confronting drug policy: illicit drugs in a free society*. Cambridge, UK: Cambridge University Press.

Grichting, E., Uchtenhagen, A., & Rehm, J. (2002). Modes and impact of coercive inpatient treatment for drug-related conditions in Switzerland. *European Addiction Research* 8, 78–83.

Hall, W. 1997. The role of legal coercion in the treatment of offenders with alcohol and heroin problems. *Australian and New Zealand Journal of Criminology* 30, 103–120.

Hall, W., & Lucke, J. (2010). Legally coerced treatment for drug using offenders: ethical and policy issues. *Crime and Justice Bulletin* 144, 1–12.

Heyman, G. (2009). *Addiction: a disorder of choice*. Cambridge, MA: Harvard University Press.

Klag, S., O'Callaghan, F., & Creed, P. (2005). The use of legal coercion in the treatment of substance abusers: an overview and critical analysis of thirty years of research. *Substance Use & Misuse* 40, 1777–1795.

Lee, N. (2015). Forcing ice users into rehab won't solve the problem – here's what we need instead. *The Conversation* [Online], 12 August. https://theconversation.com/forcing-ice-users-into-rehab-wont-solve-the-problem-heres-what-we-need-instead-45946

Leukefeld, C. G., & Tims, F. M. (Eds.) (1988). *Compulsory treatment of drug abuse: research and clinical practice*. Rockville, MD: National Institute on Drug Abuse.

Maddux, J. (1988). Clinical experience with civil commitment. In C. G. Leukefeld & F. M. Tims (Eds.), *Compulsory treatment of drug abuse: research and clinical practice*. Rockville, MD: National Institute on Drug Addiction.

Marteau, T., Ashcroft, R. E., & Oliver, A. (2009). Using financial incentives to achieve healthy behaviour. *British Medical Journal* 338, 983–985.

McLellan, A. T., Skipper, G. S., Campbell, M., & Dupont, R. L. (2008). Five year outcomes in a cohort study of physicians treated for substance use disorders in the United States. *British Medical Journal* 337, a2038.

National Research Council (2001). *Informing America's policy on illegal drugs: what we don't know keeps hurting us*. Washington, DC: National Academy Press.

New South Wales Standing Committee on Social Issues (2004). *Report on Inebriates Act 1912*. Sydney: New South Wales Parliament.

Newman, R. (1974). Involuntary treatment of drug addiction. In P. G. Bourne (Ed.), *Addiction*. New York: Academic Press.

Palm, J., & Stenius, K. (2002). Sweden: integrated compulsory treatment. *European Addiction Research* 8, 69–77.

Petry, N., Alessi, S. M., & Rush, C. (2011). Contingency management treatment for drug and alcohol use disorders. In J. S. Poland & G. Graham (Eds.), *Addiction and responsibility*. London: MIT Press.

Porter, L., Arif, A., & Curran, W. J. (1986). *The law and the treatment of drug- and alcohol- dependent persons: a comparative study of existing legislation*. Geneva: WHO.

Pritchard, E., Mugavin, J., & Swan, A. (2007). *Compulsory treatment in Australia: a discussion paper on the compulsory treatment of individuals dependent on drugs and/ or alcohol*. Canberra: Australian National Council on Drugs.

PwC's Indigenous Consulting with Menzies School of Health Research (2017). *Evaluation of the Alcohol Mandatory Treatment Program*. Darwin: Northern Territory Department of Health.

Room, R. (2007). Social policy and psychoactive substances. In D. Nutt, T. Robbins, G. Stimson, M. Ince & A. Jackson (Eds.), *Drugs and the future: brain science, addiction and society*. London: Academic Press.

Rotgers, F. (1992). Coercion in addictions treatment. In F. Rotgers, J. W. Langebucher, B. S. McCrady, W. Frankenstein & P. E. Nathan (Eds.), *Annual review of addictions research and treatment*. New York: Pergamon Press.

Satel, S., & Lilienfeld, S. O. (2014). Addiction and the brain-disease fallacy. *Frontiers in Psychiatry* 4.

Schumann, G. (2007). Okey Lecture 2006: identifying the neurobiological mechanisms of addictive behaviour. *Addiction* 102, 1689–1695.

Skene, L. (1987). An evaluation of a Victorian scheme for diversion of alcoholic and drug dependent offenders. *Australian and New Zealand Journal of Criminology* 20, 247–268.

Small, W., Kain, S., Laliberte, N., Schechter, M. T., O'Shaughnessy, M. V., & Spittal, P. M. (2005). Incarceration, addiction and harm reduction: inmates experience injecting drugs in prison. *Substance Use & Misuse* 40, 831–843.

Sullivan, M., Birkmayer, F., Boyarsky, B., Frances, R., Fromson, J., Galanter, M., Levin, F., Lewis, C., Nace, E. & Suchinsky, R. (2008). Uses of coercion in addiction treatment: clinical aspects. *American Journal on Addictions* 17, 36–47.

Szasz, T. S. (1975). *Ceremonial chemistry: the ritual persecution of drugs, addicts, and pushers*. London: Routledge.

Uhl, G. R., Drgon, T., Johnson, C., Li, C.-Y., Contoreggi, C., Hess, J., Naiman, D., & LiuQ.R.- (2008). Molecular genetics of addiction and related heritable phenotypes. *Annals of the New York Academy of Sciences 1141*, 318–381.

United Nations (1976). *The International Bill of Human Rights.* www.ohchr.org/Documents/Publications/Compilation1.1en.pdf.

UNODC (2010). *From coercion to cohesion: treating drug dependence through healthcare, not punishment: discussion paper.* Vienna: United Nations Office on Drugs and Crime.

Volkow, N., Wang, G. J., Fowler, J. S., Tomasi, D., & Baler, R. (2014). Neuroimaging of addiction. In P. Seeman & B. K. Madras (Eds.), *Imaging of the human brain in health and disease.* San Diego: Elsevier.

Volkow, N. D., Koob, G. F., & McLellan, A. T. (2016). Neurobiologic advances from the brain disease model of addiction. *New England Journal of Medicine* 374, 363–371.

Walsh, M. (2017). Amid opioid epidemic, Vivitrol finds success marketing to judges and jailers. *Yahoo News* [Online], 6 July. www.yahoo.com/news/opioid-epidemic-vivitrol-finds-success-marketing-judges-jailers-090040231.html

Webb, M. (2003). Compulsory alcoholism treatment in New South Wales. *Medicine and Law* 22, 311.

Wild, T. C. (1999). Compulsory substance-user treatment and harm reduction: a critical analysis. *Substance Use & Misuse* 34, 83–102.

Wild, T. C. (2006). Social control and coercion in addiction treatment: towards evidence-based policy and practice. *Addiction* 101, 40–49.

Wild, T. C., Newton-Taylor, B., & Alletto, R. (1998). Perceived coercion among clients entering substance abuse treatment: structural and psychological determinants. *Addictive Behaviors* 23, 81–95.

Wood, E., Montaner, J., & Kerr, T. (2005). HIV risks in incarcerated injection-drug users. *Lancet* 366, 1834–1835.

Chapter 2

Community treatment orders

The evidence and the ethical implications

Lisa Brophy, Christopher James Ryan and
Penelope Weller

Community treatment orders (CTOs) are legal orders, provided for within mental health legislation, that are made by clinicians or tribunals. CTOs set out the terms under which a person with a mental illness must accept treatment or other services while living in the community (Light et al., 2012a). The criteria for involuntary treatment differ from jurisdiction to jurisdiction, but most commonly include at least: that the person must suffer a serious mental illness; that he or she needs protections from some serious harm; that the person is refusing the treatment offered; and that an order represents the least restrictive means of providing the person with protection. Only in some jurisdictions must it also be the case that people's mental illnesses rob them of the capacity to understand or weigh relevant information when they refuse treatment (Ryan, Callaghan & Peisah, 2015). CTOs go under different names (in North America compulsory community treatment is often referred to as 'assisted outpatient treatment' or 'outpatient commitment'), and though the treatments they impose vary, in most instances they involve psychosocial interventions and medication (often delivered by long-acting injection) (Lepping & Malik, 2013; Burns & Molodynski, 2014). Non-compliance with a CTO generally results in the person being detained and either involuntarily admitted to hospital, or being given the mandated treatment before being discharged back to the community. Since their introduction, CTOs have gradually become a standard feature of contemporary mental health care internationally (Brophy & McDermott, 2003; Burns & Molodynski, 2014; Light, 2014).

Community treatment order legislation emerged in tandem with the demise of large stand-alone psychiatric institutions and flourished in response to community concerns about suicide and violence (Behnke, 1999; Muijen, 1996). It was hoped that CTOs might prevent relapse, minimise repeated, 'revolving door' admissions (Dawson, 2008; Elbogen & Tomkins, 2000) and provide families and carers of persons with severe mental illness with much needed support (Power, 1999). Whether CTOs have actually achieved these outcomes is increasingly doubted, and there have been recent calls for them to be abandoned or dramatically scaled back (Callaghan & Newton-Howes,

2017; Newton-Howes & Ryan, 2017; United Nations, 2017). Furthermore, CTOs are seen by some to be incompatible with human rights obligations and to hinder, rather than assist, the recovery of people with mental illness.

This chapter attempts to make sense of the controversy surrounding CTOs by considering three aspects of their use: their compatibility with human rights; their efficacy; and their impact on individuals and healthcare systems. We conclude by briefly examining some alternatives to CTOs.

Background and the international context

Community treatment orders have been adopted in the vast majority of the United States, all jurisdictions in Australia, New Zealand, England, Wales, Scotland, Israel and nine provinces in Canada (Light et al., 2012b). They exist in Norway, Sweden and Denmark, but are not a common feature of legislation in continental Europe (Churchill et al., 2007; Ramon, 2006; Rugkåsa, 2016). In contrast to the United States and the United Kingdom, where the implementation of CTOs has occurred in the context of considerable controversy, stakeholders in Australia, Canada and New Zealand generally reacted positively to their introduction (Dawson, 2005; Gibbs et al., 2005; Gibbs, Dawson, & Mullen, 2006; O'Brien & Farrell, 2004; O'Reilly et al., 2006).

Are community treatment orders compatible with human rights?

The degree to which CTOS are compatible with human rights is hotly disputed. While some commentators have argued that CTOs contravene human rights on the basis of their being compulsory treatment (Minkowitz, 2006), others claim CTOs provide a vehicle for the realisation of a patient's positive rights to care and treatment (Dawson, 2005). The advent of the *Convention on the Rights of Person with Disabilities* (CRPD) (United Nations, 2007), the international human rights instrument governing the rights of people with disabilities, has changed the contours of the human rights debate, but not dampened the controversy (Freeman et al., 2015; Maylea, 2016).

While its implications for mental health law remain unresolved, it is clear is that the CRPD marks a significant turning point in the international human rights framework. It responds to the lived experience of people with disabilities by adopting a clear emphasis on equality, nondiscrimination and social inclusion, and a new approach to the notion of equal access to goods and services, particularly the social, environmental and material determinants of health (Weller, 2010). Article 12 requires equal recognition before the law; Article 17 requires respect for physical and mental integrity; Article 25 protects the right to health by privileging the right to control one's health and body. The CRPD rejects the traditional position in the law that those who lack capacity should be subject to 'best interests' determinations. Rather, it requires a radical reinterpretation of participation in decision-making that asserts that people with disabilities be at the heart of decision-making inter-actions which respect the person's rights, will and preferences (United Nations, 2014). The CRPD committee asserts that in cases where the wishes of the person are not known, decisions should be made on the basis of the 'best interpretation of will and preferences' (United Nations, 2014, para 21). In short, the CRPD recognises that human rights principles do not insist on independent decision-making, but focus on the quality of the interaction between people with disability. In doing so the CRPD creates a new approach to decision-making in health. While the practices that will support that approach are yet to emerge, it is clear that CTOs in their standard form are inconsistent with international human rights principles (Newton-Howes & Ryan, 2017).

McSherry (2008) argues human rights protection of the right to physical and mental integrity in the CRPD is unlikely to completely overturn invo-luntary treatment, but will enable greater restriction on 'unbeneficial and overly intrusive treatment' (p. 122). If CTOs are to be appropriately limited, rather than abolished, the question of whether they 'work' remains pertinent.

Do community treatment orders work?

What we mean by 'work' and how to judge this

Questions about the efficacy of a particular treatment (or element in treat-ment delivery) are common in medicine. One way to pose such questions is to consider whether people afforded an intervention will benefit from it, but this question raises two further issues.

The first issue arises from the fact that no treatment will benefit everyone who gets it: even if some people benefit from being subject to a CTO, others will derive no benefit. The second issue is a reflection on what we mean by 'benefit' and how that can be measured. Ultimately, we are interested in whether the person's life is better on the treatment, but there are two serious problems with examining benefit in this sense. First, general well-being is essentially a subjective measure. Whether or how a person's life is 'improved' will be interpreted differently by each person. Second, as so many factors influence well-being, it is hard to know to what extent the treatment of inter-est contributed to any improvement seen. The latter problem is particularly significant when the supposed benefits of treatment have taken months or even years to manifest. For these reasons, quantitative researchers tend to avoid measures of general well-being, and focus instead on outcomes that are more circumscribed, easier to measure and directly related to the intervention.

Randomised controlled trials of community treatment order effectiveness

The studies that are usually regarded as most likely to yield meaningful results are randomised controlled trials (RCTs). RCTs are studies that randomly place some participants into one group that gets the intervention and others into a group that does not. The outcomes of the two groups are compared at the end of the study. The idea is that the randomisation will render the two groups roughly the same, with the only real difference between them being whether patients got the intervention. Any 'improvements' observed in one group are then attributed to the intervention.

Three RCTs have tested the effectiveness of CTOs. Before discussing their results, it must be noted that all had significant limitations, both in terms of the way they were conducted and in terms of the extent to which their results can be generalised to other populations.

The first RCT of CTOs was conducted in New York State in the 1990s (Steadman et al., 2001). It was a state-sanctioned pilot program to gauge the effectiveness of what would become known as Kendra's law (*New York Mental Hygiene Law* § 9.60). The study had multiple problems. It was small, with only 142 participants – fewer than half of those eligible for enrolment in the study. The study ran for 12 months, but 45% of participants dropped out before the end. It was not clear to what extent the research protocol was adhered to and there was confusion among staff and patients about who was, and who was not, on a CTO. Finally, no non-compliant patient was ever made subject to the 'pickup procedure' that the law enabled, which would have seen the patient brought forcibly back to hospital for treatment.

The second study, based in North Carolina, was conducted over the same period as the New York study and had a very similar design (Swartz et al., 1999). It was larger than the New York study, following 264 patients, and had a much smaller dropout rate. The North Carolina statute allowed an order to be made for a maximum of 90 days, but the orders were usually made for only 30 to 60 days *(NC Gen Stat* § 122C-271). Both US studies excluded patients with a history of violence, and this, together with the unique characteristics of the US population and health system, mean that it is hard to translate their findings into day-to-day practice outside the United States.

The OCTET study (Burns et al., 2013) was much larger than either of the US studies; it randomised 366 patients to either a CTO or a control group who were given leave under section 17 of the UK *Mental Health Act*. Section 17 allowed patients to leave the hospital for days, or even months, while still subject to recall. The OCTET study also had problems. For example, although the length of initial compulsory outpatient treatment differed significantly between the two groups, with a median length of 183 days in the CTO group compared with eight days in the control group, patients in the control group eventually averaged four months on some form of compulsory treatment. Consequently, the intervention and control groups may not have been treated that differently. Additionally, the study protocol allowed treating clinicians to later make treatment decisions independent of the initial randomisation, and as a result around a fifth of patients in both arms swapped treatments.

The brief reviews above lists reasons to doubt the overall validity and generalisability of the three RCTs. With that significant caveat in mind, what did they find?

The three RCTs examined a variety of outcomes. All examined whether CTOs led to an avoidance of readmission to hospital. The New York and North Carolina studies examined compliance with medication, avoidance of arrest, avoidance of homelessness and whether there was an improvement in subjective well-being or quality of life. The OCTET study also examined whether CTOs led to fewer days in hospital or improvement in symptoms and general function. The North Carolina study also examined if the patients on CTOs were less likely to be the victims of crime. Of all these potential outcomes across the three studies, the only outcome to reach statistical significance was the last – the avoidance of victimisation in the North Carolina study. This disappointing lack of positive effect remained even when the results of the individually small studies were combined via meta-analysis (Kisely & Campbell, 2014).

Other quantitative studies of the effectiveness of community treatment orders

Although RCTs are generally regarded as the gold standard in determining whether an intervention is effective, they are not always the best method of approaching effectiveness questions. When researching CTOs, it is very difficult to recruit large numbers of participants to an RCT. If the benefits of a CTO are relatively small, they may simply not become apparent if studies can only enrol a few hundred people. There may also be ethical difficulties with randomising some patients to CTOs and others not, which may explain why the US studies excluded patients with a history of violence.

These considerations have led some researchers to turn to epidemiological and case-control studies to try to determine the effectiveness of CTOs. These studies typically use large government databases to retrospectively compare the outcomes of larger numbers of patients, some of whom have been subject to CTOs and others not. Studies of this sort cannot be randomised, so researchers must make some effort to try to match the patients who have been placed on CTOs with those who have not. The aim is to try to compare like with like – to make the argument that the only real difference between the patients who were placed on a CTO and those that were not was the CTO.

There have been more than 90 of these types of studies and several detailed reviews (Churchill et al., 2007; Maughan et al., 2014; Rugkåsa, Dawson, & Burns, 2014). The studies have examined a range of possible benefits of

CTOs, including a decreased rate of readmission to hospital; a decrease in the number of readmissions; fewer days in hospital; improved social function; community service use; and a reduction in all-cause mortality. Unfortunately, an overview of all these studies reveals inconsistent and conflicting results. In some studies, the changes in some of the potential indicators of CTO benefit reach statistical significance, but in others they do not. In some studies, CTOs appear to improve these indicators, and in other studies, the indicators decline.

One of the most reported indicators is the rate of readmission to hospital, which was examined in 22 studies. Thirteen studies suggested that CTOs decreased the rate of readmission of people subject to them, but four studies suggested the rate of readmission *increased* when CTOs were used. The remaining five studies mirrored the findings of the RCTs, suggesting CTOs made no difference to the rate of readmission (Rugkåsa et al., 2014). To further complicate matters, sometimes the decrease in readmission only occurred after a person was on a CTO for six months, a finding that may be the result of a biased process, as CTOs are often renewed at around six months and it may be that some clinicians will only renew a CTO when it is felt that the person subject to it is benefiting from it. Even more confusingly, it is not clear that more readmissions can properly be regarded as a bad outcome. Some authors argue that, on the contrary, early readmission before the patient gets very sick is a *good* thing and may lead to less time in hospital overall (Segal & Burgess, 2006), though that line of thought is somewhat undermined by a similar examination of studies that examine the effect that CTOs have on the number of days spent in hospital, which also have inconsistent results (Rugkåsa et al., 2014).

One of the most robust findings came from a Western Australian cohort, where it was found that people placed on a CTO appeared to benefit from a significant reduction in all-cause mortality (Kisely et al., 2013). However, in this study, and in several of the other positive studies, the authors speculate that the benefit was not due to the coercive effect of CTOs per se, but rather to the increased contact with health professionals associated with CTO use. The deaths in the West Australian study were primarily from physical illnesses such as cancer, cardiovascular disease or diseases of the central nervous system, and the improvement associated with CTO use disappeared when adjusted for increased outpatient and community contacts with psychiatric services.

If, to the extent that CTOs are effective, they are only effective because they provide a key to gaining access to a service that people could, or should, have had available anyway – perhaps by influencing healthcare staff to provide a better service – then they are not being effective via their power to compel and, in a real sense, are not really effective at all.

The latest round of large cohort studies, which use new techniques to match those who were subject to CTOs with those who were not, appear to be finding more robust evidence of efficacy, at least with respect to decreased admissions. However, these studies suggest that the benefits of CTOs are modest at best. For example, one recent study, conducted in Australia, found that CTOs could decrease the number of readmissions, but the number of people that needed to be subject to a CTO to prevent one person from any readmission over a three-year period was 48 (Harris, Garside, & Sara, 2014). Even if one person will benefit from a CTO, it is hard ethically to justify forcing treatment upon 48 others who will not.

Taking account of all the available quantitative studies conducted to date (RCTs, cohort and epidemiological studies), there is little or nothing to support a conclusion that CTOs are effective via their ability to compel individuals to accept treatment without consent. Such is the state of the evidence, the authors of one systematic review conclude: 'there is now robust evidence in the literature that CTOs have *no* significant effects on hospitalisation and other service use outcomes' (Maughan et al., 2014). Though arguably this conclusion goes beyond the state of the evidence to date, exactly when one should deem a lack of evidence of effectiveness as evidence of a lack of effectiveness is an issue upon which reasonable minds will differ.

Evaluating the wider impact of community treatment orders

Debates about the use and consequences of community treatment orders

While some of the literature surrounding CTOs contends that they are inherently coercive and therefore unacceptable, others assert that the experience of coercion, even though it may be distressing, needs to be weighed against the potential benefits of CTOs (Mfoafo-M'Carthy & Williams, 2010). Studies attempting to assess the degree of perceived coercion experienced by people on CTOs have produced mixed results (Kisely & Campbell, 2014). Some have argued that the coercive impact of CTOs has been exaggerated (O'Reilly et al., 2006), while others have stated that at least some people are 'totally humiliated' by all forms of coercion in psychiatric care, including forced medication (Nyttingnes, Ruud & Rugkåsa, 2016).

There are now many studies suggesting that CTOs are perceived as important in assisting people with mental illness to gain access to services for continuity of care or when in crisis. In these studies, CTOs are understood as an expression of the commitment of the service to the person on a CTO (Light et al., 2017). Swartz et al. (1999), for example, conclude that a CTO 'works when it represents a reciprocal commitment by community programmes to provide sustained and intensive treatment to patients under court orders' (p. 1974). In these studies CTOs are, rather pragmatically, considered positively because they enable continuity of care.

Nevertheless, the imperative to ensure adequate follow-up of people on CTOs creates significant problems for service providers and may generate unintended consequences (Brophy & McDermott, 2003; Light et al., 2017). For example, Power (1999) found that while there is considerable support from service providers for CTOs in well-targeted situations, CTOs may act as a further deterrent to treatment compliance when poorly targeted. Whether or not that is true, CTOs are difficult to administer with homeless or itinerant people – those most at risk of becoming unwell.

CTOs have also been associated with a net-widening effect that occurs after their introduction (Geller et al., 2006), where the use of CTOs expands beyond those initially targeted to other groups, such as those experiencing only their first episode of illness (Morandi et al., 2017), or to women with less severe illness or less impoverished social circumstances (Brophy, Reece, & McDermott, 2006). A related concern is a potential 'lobster pot effect' (Morandi, 2016), in which there is a low threshold for being placed on a CTO, but a higher threshold for having it removed. Carney (2003) argues there is a growing, invisible, marginalised group of people in the community who experience significant curtailment to their human rights and are at risk of further stigma and discrimination.

Key stakeholder perspectives

Another way of examining the effect of CTOs is to consider the 'lived experience' of the people involved in their implementation, such as those who have been on a CTO, their families or carers, and service providers (mainly psychiatrists). There is a consistency in relation to qualitative findings across jurisdictions and over time, suggesting considerable similarities in the lived experience of people subject to CTOs (Churchill et al., 2007; Corring, O'Reilly, & Sommerdyck, 2017). In some studies, CTOs are described positively, offering 'comparative liberty'. People on them report that it is better to be on a CTO than to be in hospital, gaol or subject to other forms of coercion (Corring et al., 2017; McDonnell & Bartholomew, 1997). Some people have been observed to request a CTO in order to feel safe, have a boundary or avoid the potential of being overlooked or abandoned by service providers (Corring et al., 2017; Dawson, 2005; McDonnell & Bartholomew, 1997). Others appear to be simultaneously resisting and accepting orders (Canvin, Bartlett, & Pinfold, 2002; Gibbs et al., 2005). Corring et al. (2017) found that people are sometimes ambivalent about 'balancing acceptance of enforced treatment with feelings of increased wellness' (p. 4).

Lived experience research in New Zealand (Gibbs et al., 2005), Canada (O'Reilly et al., 2006), the United States (Swartz et al., 2003; Wales & Hiday, 2006) and Australia (Brophy & Ring, 2004) highlights the issue of people 'not feeling heard' about medication preferences and side effects. Being heard, respected and receiving high-quality treatment in the context of genuinely helpful relationships is commonly viewed as important, although deficiencies are often identified (Corring et al., 2017). Many people on CTOs see medication adherence as their main rationale. People in these studies appear to be engaged in active evaluation of their care and express concerns about the poor standard of care they are receiving (Canvin et al., 2002; Corrigan & Liberman, 1990). For some this might be described as concerns about a lack of reciprocity. Reciprocity would require people on CTOs to receive a level of service, treatment and care commensurate with the loss of liberty they experience (Bartlett & Sandland, 2007); hence deficiencies in service delivery are potentially reframed as a human rights issue (Light et al., 2017).

Lived experience research also reveals an emphasis on safety and security (Churchill et al., 2007). CTOs have been compared to having an insurance policy or safety net, particularly in relation to ensuring that services are accessible and cannot be withdrawn (Light et al., 2017). People who view CTOs in this light appreciate that services are obliged to provide them with care, and family and carers are relieved that they are receiving assistance in helping their loved ones (Corring et al., 2017; Mullen, Dawson, & Gibbs, 2006).

Corring et al. (2017) identify CTOs as being associated with difficult relationships with clinicians, even though some studies have found fewer negative effects. In New Zealand, it was suggested that CTOs offered, at least in the long term, the possibility of enhancing the relationship – through enabling engagement and providing a structure or framework for difficult conversations to occur (Gibbs et al., 2006). Service providers do express concerns about the difficulties in balancing the care and control dimensions of their practice when implementing CTOs (Churchill et al., 2007). Key stakeholders also often have poor awareness about their rights and responsibilities and the powers contained in CTO legislation (Atkinson et al., 2002; Rolfe, Sheehan, & Davidson, 2008).

Alternatives to community treatment orders

In response to doubts about the clinical efficacy of CTOs and the wide impacts of a mental health system based on coercion, it is important to consider whether there are alternatives to CTOs (Nagra et al., 2016). Szmukler (2015) argues that, in the context of increased use of involuntary care without adequate evidence of its effectiveness, and international human rights obligations, all efforts should be made to reduce the use of coercion, including CTOs.

Many alternative approaches and interventions have been proposed. Some have called for far greater emphasis on whether a person's ability to competently refuse treatment has been affected by their illness. Dawson and Szmukler (2006) have long advocated the abandonment of specific mental health legislation, favouring the adoption of legislation that covers all people with impaired decision-making capacity, whether this is due to mental or physical illness. Others have insisted that CTO legislation should not allow the forced treatment of people whose refusal of psychiatric treatment is competent (Newton-Howes & Ryan, 2017). Still others suggest that people with lived experience of mental illness should be an integral part of legislated panels that review a person's decision-making capacity (Munetz & Frese, 2001).

While CTOs offer one way of increasing a person's acceptance of treatment in the community, there is a paucity of research on other, less coercive methods of achieving the same end. For example, simply increasing the intensity of therapeutic contact with a person in the community improves outcomes without the need for coercion, but this is yet to be compared to CTOs in efficacy studies (Kisely & Campbell, 2014). The availability of housing is also a form of leverage into treatment that has rarely been the subject of research (Monahan et al., 2005).

Advance directives and advance statements are additional mechanisms by which people with mental illness can set out their treatment preferences when well, so that they may inform treatment decisions if they later lose decision-making capacity. These and other ways of supporting a person's decision-making are favoured by many service users (Henderson et al., 2008). While the efficacy of these tools is only now beginning to be examined, de Jong et al. (2016) conclude that there is greater evidence for the effectiveness of advance directives in reducing compulsory admission than there is for CTOs.

Conclusion

The *Convention on the Rights of Persons with Disabilities* has raised the stakes on the human rights credentials of CTOs. Moreover, an analysis of the efficacy of CTOs reveals mixed evidence at best and a likelihood that any positive effects are probably small. The utilisation of CTOs seems influenced by more than just the needs of the people subject to them. Social and structural issues are also being played out in their existence and implementation. Nonetheless, CTOs are now embedded in the mental health care systems of many jurisdictions and impact on how those systems operate. They may be encouraging an increased reliance on coercion to achieve compliance with treatment, and sometimes appear to do naught but facilitate access to necessary care and treatment. The evidence about their effectiveness from both qualitative and quantitative research is mixed and does not appear to be the main driver of practice or policy change.

The high and increasing use of CTOs is a problem. Calls for a moratorium or at least a dramatic reduction of their use ought to be heeded (Burns & Molodynski, 2014; Callaghan & Newton-Howes, 2017; Newton-Howes & Ryan, 2017). Non-coercive alternatives such as decision-making supports and improvements in treatment and service provision must be explored.

References

Atkinson, J. M., Garner, H. C., Gilmour, W. H., & Dyer, J. A. T. (2002). Changes to leave of absence in Scotland: the views of patients. *Journal of Forensic Psychiatry*, 13, 315–328.

Bartlett, P., & Sandland, R. (2007). *Mental health law: policy and practice*. Oxford: Oxford University Press.

Behnke, S. H. (1999). Outpatient commitment laws: forcing mentally ill patients to take their medication. *Lahey Clinic Medical Ethics Newsletter* 4, 8.

Brophy, L. & McDermott, F. (2003). What's driving involuntary treatment in the community? The social, policy, legal and ethical context. *Australasian Psychiatry* 11, S84–S88.

Brophy, L., & Ring, D. (2004). The efficacy of involuntary treatment in the community. *Social Work in Mental Health* 2, 157–174.

Brophy, L. M., Reece, J. E., & McDermott, F. (2006). A cluster analysis of people on Community Treatment Orders in Victoria, Australia. *International Journal of Law and Psychiatry* 29, 469–481.

Burns, T., & Molodynski, A. (2014). Community treatment orders: background and implications of the OCTET trial. *Psychiatric Bulletin* 38(4), 197.

Burns, T., Rugkåsa, J., Molodynski, A., Dawson, J., Yeeles, K., Vazquez-Montes, M., Voysey, M., Sinclair, J., & Priebe, S. (2013). Community treatment orders for patients with psychosis (OCTET): a randomised controlled trial. *Lancet* 381, 1627–1633.

Callaghan, S., & Newton-Howes, G. (2017). Coercive community treatment in mental health: an idea whose time has passed? *Journal of Law and Medicine* 24, 900–914.

Canvin, K., Bartlett, A., & Pinfold, V. (2002). A 'bittersweet pill to swallow': learning from mental health service users' responses to compulsory community care in England *Health and Social Care in the Community* 10, 361–369.

Carney, T. (2003). Mental health law in postmodern society: time for new paradigms? *Psychiatry, Psychology and Law* 10, 12–32.

Churchill, R., Owen, G., Singh, S., & Hotopf, M. (2007). *International experiences of using community treatment orders*. London: Department of Health.

Corrigan, P. W., & Liberman, R. P. (1990). From noncompliance to collaboration in the treatment of schizophrenia. *Hospital and Community Psychiatry* 41, 1203–1211.

Corring, D., O'Reilly, R., & Sommerdyck, C. (2017). A systematic review of the views and experiences of subjects of community treatment orders. *International Journal of Law and Psychiatry* 52, 74–80. doi:10.1016/j.ijlp.2017.03.002

Dawson, J. (2005). *Community treatment orders: international comparisons*. Dunedin: Otago University Print.

Dawson, J. (2008). Community treatment orders and human rights. *Law in Context* 26, 148–159.

Dawson, J., & Szmukler, G. (2006). Fusion of mental health and incapacity legislation. *British Journal of Psychiatry* 188, 504–509.

de Jong, M. H., Kamperman, A. M., Oorschot, M., Priebe, S., Bramer, W., Van De Sande, R., Van Gool, A. R., & Mulder, C. L. (2016). Interventions to reduce compulsory psychiatric admissions: a systematic review and meta-analysis. *JAMA Psychiatry* 73, 657–664.

Elbogen, E. B., & Tomkins, A. J. (2000). From the psychiatric hospital to the community: integrating conditional release and contingency management. *Behaviour Sciences and the Law* 18, 427–444.

Freeman, M. C., Kolappa, K., De Almeida, J. M. C., Kleinman, A., Makhashvili, N., Phakathi, S., Saraceno, B., & Thornicroft, G. (2015). Reversing hard won victories in the name of human rights: a critique of the General Comment on Article 12 of the UN Convention on the Rights of Persons with Disabilities. *Lancet Psychiatry* 2, 844–850.

Geller, J. L., Fisher, W. H., Grudzinskas, A. J., Jr., Clayfield, J. C., & Lawlor, T. (2006). Involuntary outpatient treatment as 'desintitutionalized coercion': the net-widening concerns. *International Journal of Law and Psychiatry* 29, 551–562.

Gibbs, A., Dawson, J., Ansley, C., & Mullen, R. (2005). How patients in New Zealand view community treatment orders. *Journal of Mental Health* 14, 357–368.

Gibbs, A., Dawson, J., & Mullen, R. (2006). Community treatment orders for people with serious mental illness: a New Zealand study. *British Journal of Social Work* 36, 1085–1100.

Harris, A. W., Garside, J., & Sara, G. (2014). Do community treatment orders keep people out of hospital? The influence of the level of community care. *Schizophrenia Research* 153, S321.

Henderson, C., Swanson, J. W., Szmukler, G., Thornicroft, G. & Zinkler, M. (2008). A typology of advance statements in mental health care. *Psychiatric Services* 59, 63–71.

Kisely, S., Preston, N., Xiao, J., Lawrence, D., Louise, S., & Crowe, E. (2013). Reducing all-cause mortality among patients with psychiatric disorders: a population-based study. *Canadian Medical Association Journal* 185, E50–56.

Kisely, S. R., & Campbell, L. A. (2014). Compulsory community and involuntary outpatient treatment for people with severe mental disorders (Review). *Cochrane Database of Systematic Reviews*, CD004408.

Lepping, P., & Malik, M. (2013). Community treatment orders: current practice and a framework to aid clinicians. *The Psychiatrist* 37, 54–57.

Light, E. (2014). The epistemic challenges of CTOs: commentary on … community treatment orders. *Psychiatric Bulletin* 38(1), 6–8.

Light, E., Robertson, M., Ryan, C. J., & Kerridge, I. H. (2012a). Out of sight, out of mind: making involuntary community treatment visible in the mental health system. *Medical Journal of Australia* 196, 591–593.

Light, E. M., Kerridge, I. H., Ryan, C. J., & Robertson, M. (2012b). Community treatment orders: rates and patterns of use. *Australasian Psychiatry* 20, 478–482.

Light, E. M., Robertson, M. D., Boyce, P., Carney, T., Rosen, A., Cleary, M., Hunt, G. E., O'Connor, N., Ryan, C. J., & Kerridge, I. H. (2017). How shortcomings in the mental health system affect the use of involuntary community treatment orders. *Australian Health Review* 41, 351–356.

Maughan, D., Molodynski, A., Rugkåsa, J., & Burns, T. (2014). A systematic review of the effect of community treatment orders on service use. *Social Psychiatry and Psychiatric Epidemiology* 49, 651–663.

Maylea, C. H. (2016). A rejection of involuntary treatment in mental health social work. *Ethics and Social Welfare*, 1–17.

McDonnell, E., & Bartholomew, T. (1997). Community treatment orders in Victoria: Emergent issues and anomalies. *Psychiatry, Psychology and Law* 4, 25–36.

McSherry, B. (2008). Protecting the integrity of the person: developing limitations on involuntary treatment. *Law in Context* 26, 111–124.

Mfoafo-M'Carthy, M., & Williams, C. C. (2010). Coercion and community treatment orders (CTOs): one step forward, two steps back? *Canadian Journal of Community Mental Health* 29, 69–80.

Minkowitz, T. (2006). *No-force advocacy by users and survivors of psychiatry.* Wellington: Mental Health Commission.

Monahan, J., Redlich, A. D., Swanson, J., Robbins, P. C., Appelbaum, P. S., Petrila, J., Steadman, H. J., Swartz, M., Angell, B., & McNiel, D. E. (2005). Use of leverage to improve adherence to psychiatric treatment in the community. *Psychiatric Services* 56, 37–44.

Morandi, S. (2016). Descriptive and epidemiological studies. In A. Molodynski, J. Rugkåsa & T. Burns (Eds.), *Coercion in community mental health care: international perspectives.* Oxford: Oxford University Press.

Morandi, S., Golay, P., Lambert, M., Schimmelmann, B. G., McGorry, P. D., Cotton, S. M., & Conus, P. (2017). Community treatment order: identifying the need for more evidence based justification of its use in first episode psychosis patients. *Schizophrenia Research* 185, 67–72. doi:10.1016/j.schres.2016.12.022

Muijen, M. (1996). Scare in the community: Britain in moral panic. In T. Heller, J. Reynolds, R. Gomm, R. Muston. & S. Pattison (Eds.), *Mental health matters: a reader.* London: Macmillan.

Mullen, R., Dawson, J., & Gibbs, A. (2006). Dilemmas for clinicians in use of community treatment orders. *International Journal of Law and Psychiatry* 29, 535–550.

Munetz, M. R., & Frese, F., J. (2001). Getting ready for recovery: reconciling mandatory treatment with the recovery revision. *Psychiatric Rehabilitation Journal* 25, 35–42.

Nagra, M. K., Pillinger, T., Prata-Ribeiro, H., Khazaal, Y., & Molodynski, A. (2016). Community Treatment Orders – a pause for thought. *Asian Journal of Psychiatry* 24, 1–4.

Newton-Howes, G., & Ryan, C. J. (2017). The use of CTOs in competent patients is not justified. *British Journal of Psychiatry* 210, 311–312.

Nyttingnes, O., Ruud, T., & Rugkåsa, J. (2016). 'It's unbelievably humiliating' – patients' expressions of negative effects of coercion in mental health care. *International Journal of Law and Psychiatry* 49, 147–153.

O'Brien, A. M. A.- & Farrell, S. J. (2004). Community treatment orders: Profile of a Canadian experience. *Canadian Journal of Psychiatry, 50*, 27–30.

O'Reilly, R. L., Keegan, D. L., Corring, D., Shrikhande, S., & Natarajan, D. (2006). A qualitative analysis of the use of community treatment orders in Saskatchewan. *International Journal of Law and Psychiatry* 29, 516–524.

Power, P. (1999). Community treatment orders: The Australian experience. *The Journal of Forensic Psychiatry, 10*, 9–15.

Ramon, S. (2006). Risk avoidance and risk taking in mental health social work. In L. Sapouna & P. Herrmann (Eds.), *Knowledge in mental health: reclaiming the social.* New York: Nova Science.

Rolfe, T., Sheehan, B., & Davidson, R. (2008). Are consumers on community treatment orders informed of their legal and human rights? A West Australian study. *International Journal of Mental Health Nursing* 17, 36–43.

Rugkåsa, J. (2016). Effectiveness of community treatment orders: the international evidence. *Canadian Journal of Psychiatry* 61, 15–24.

Rugkåsa, J., Dawson, J., & Burns, T. (2014). CTOs: what is the state of the evidence? *Social Psychiatry and Psychiatric Epidemiology* 49, 1861–1871.

Ryan, C. J., Callaghan, S., & Peisah, C. (2015). The capacity to refuse psychiatric treatment – a guide to the law for clinicians and tribunal members. *Australian & New Zealand Journal of Psychiatry, 49*, 324–333.

Segal, S. P., & Burgess, P. M. (2006). Conditional release: a less restrictive alternative to hospitalization? *Psychiatric Services* 57, 1600–1606.

Steadman, H. J., Gounis, K., Dennis, D., Hopper, K., Roche, B., Swartz, M., & Robbins, P. C. (2001). Assessing the New York City Involuntary Outpatient Commitment Pilot Program. *Psychiatric Services* 52, 330–336.

Swartz, M. S., Swanson, J. W., Wagner, H. R., Burns, B. J., Hiday, V. A., & Borum, R. (1999). Can involuntary outpatient commitment reduce hospital recidivism? Findings from a randomized trial with severely mentally ill individuals. *American Journal of Psychiatry* 156, 1968–1975.

Swartz, M. S., Swanson, J. W., Wagner, H. R., Hannon, M. J., Burns, B. J., & Shumway, M. (2003). Assessment of four stakeholder groups' preferences concerning outpatient commitment for persons with schizophrenia. *American Journal of Psychiatry* 160, 1139–1146.

Szmukler, G. (2015). Compulsion and 'coercion' in mental health care. *World Psychiatry* 14, 259–261.

United Nations. (2007). *Convention on the Rights of Persons with Disabilities.* Geneva: UN Doc: A/RES/61/106

United Nations. (2014). *Committee on the Rights of Persons with Disabilities. General Comment No. 1. Article 12: Equal Recognition before the Law, CRPD/C/11/4 (2014).*

United Nations. (2017). *Report of the Special Rapporteur on the Right of Everyone to the Enjoyment of the Highest Attainable Standard of Physical and Mental Health, Thirty-fifth session, A/HRC/35/21.*

Wales, H. W., & Hiday, V. A. (2006). PLC or TLC: is outpatient commitment the/an answer? *International Journal of Law and Psychiatry* 29, 451–468.

Weller, P. (2010). The right to health. The Convention of the Rights of Persons with Disabilities. *Alternative Law Journal* 35, 66–71.

Legislation

Mental Health Act 1983 (UK)
New York Mental Hygiene Law § 9.60
NC Gen Stat § 122C-271

The ambivalence of addiction medicine to the concept of involuntary treatment is costing patients dearly

Robert Batey

The idea of forcing treatment onto unwilling patients is not a popular one. Whether the treatment is mandated (court ordered) or involuntary (if the individual lacks capacity to give consent), there is significant resistance to the concept of compulsory treatments. Where data exist to demonstrate the efficacy and public health benefit of some mandated treatment (e.g., compulsory treatment of tuberculosis, vaccination programs for a wide range of infections), there are those in the community who believe the mandatory nature of even these programs is unacceptable (Bärnighausen et al., 2014; Galanakis et al., 2013; Randall, Curran & Omer, 2013). This chapter deals with the controversial area of addiction medicine, a field in which treatments are far less efficacious than those for infectious diseases, and in which the underlying condition poses a less acute risk to the individual but not necessarily the community. Compulsory treatment for dependent patients is highly controversial (Birgin et al., 2013; Klag, O'Callaghan & Creed, 2005; Wu, 2013). Nevertheless, in this chapter I argue that there is a need for greater use of it for selected individuals and under specific conditions. The argument is based on several observations:

- dependency is still poorly understood and our treatments are of limited efficacy;
- patient drop-out rates from all forms of treatment in the addiction medicine field are high (residential rehab, outpatient clinics, opioid substitution therapy programs) but those who persist in treatment do better than those who drop out (Bell et al., 2009; Burns et al., 2009; Grahn et al., 2015; Padyab, Grahn & Lundgren, 2015); and
- continued drug use (particularly alcohol) contributes to ongoing tissue damage in multiple organ systems to the detriment of the individual, their relationships and the community. Continued alcohol use may further impair capacity to make rational decisions.

Involuntary and or mandated treatment programs for drug dependence have been employed in Australia, the US and UK, and in Asian countries, including Hong Kong, Viet Nam and Malaysia, for many years. However, documentation and evaluation of these programs and their outcomes is poor (Klag et al., 2005; Werb et al., 2016). Thirty years of personal clinical experience affirm that when the option of mandated or involuntary treatment is presented to patients dispassionately and factually, many accept the option as a last but potentially positive resort. I argue that involuntary or mandated treatment can be justified, but only if programs produce much-needed data on efficacy. This will be achieved if:

- mandated treatment is used for specifically selected, high-risk dependent patients, before irreversible organ damage has been sustained; and
- units offering mandated treatments are funded adequately and compelled to monitor their program delivery, content and the outcomes achieved.

In this chapter, I make the case for mandated treatment being a part of the list of potential options for clinicians dealing with dependent users of alcohol or other drugs by:

- discussing 'acceptable' forms of involuntary or mandated therapy in general and in the setting of mental illness;
- presenting two case histories to highlight clinical issues involved in the discussion of involuntary treatment, including:
  a   the apparent willingness of opponents to mandated treatment to see imprisonment as an acceptable alternative; and
  b   the need to consider the destructive effects of waiting for a patient to reach 'rock bottom' or to reach the right point on the 'cycle of change';
- examining the reality of progressive organ damage (brain damage in particular) in those who continue to use alcohol and, to a lesser degree, other drugs of dependence;
- seeking evidence for efficacy from existing mandated programs, particularly in Australia, that deal with severely drug dependent individuals; and
- summarising the guidelines that should underpin the establishment of any future mandatory treatment facilities for dependent individuals.

'Acceptable' involuntary or mandated treatments

Imposing the will of the State or of a managing clinician on a patient against their will is seen by many as unethical and wrong even when the intervention is of proven benefit, as with vaccination (Bärnighausen et al., 2014; Galanakis et al., 2013), but as in any heated discussion, exceptions are made (Birgin et al., 2013; Halem, 1997). For example, in contrast to negative attitudes towards mandated treatment for chronic conditions such as mental health disorders and dependency, cardiopulmonary resuscitation (CPR) – frequently administered by members of the public (trained and untrained), before anyone can provide consent – is widely acceptable, despite the fact that CPR undertaken outside a hospital has a survival rate of less than 15% (Girotra et al., 2016). Perhaps the fact that death is nearly inevitable in this situation alters thinking about ethical requirements. Severe drug dependency, the subject of this chapter, is less 'dramatic', less understood, and while the mortality from this condition is high, it is not inevitable. This reality may explain why there is public acceptance of an intervention such as CPR, which does save some lives, but ongoing rejection of the fundamental concept of mandating a person to receive treatment for a more chronic condition.

Involuntary treatment in the mental health specialty

For decades, persons suffering from mental health conditions have been subjected to involuntary treatments when their illness has threatened their safety (Baur, 2013; Laffey 2003; Neugebauer, 1979). Treatments included incarceration in 'mental health facilities', medications, electroconvulsive or insulin-shock therapy, and outpatient compulsory community treatment orders. Baur (2013) helpfully describes the shift from a legal approach to mental disease in the 1700s in the UK to our present situation, in which the medical model of mental health prevails (in the West, at least). Many applaud that shift but insist involuntary treatment, under a medical model, impinges on an individual's rights. Indeed it does, but if its application improves the individual's health, an argument can be made that such treatment is worthwhile. In attempting to provide more patients with greater freedom by releasing them from institutional care and allowing them a role in deciding on treatment options, we have gone too far (see Chapter 2, this volume). Mental health patients freed from institutional care and living in community facilities now risk incarceration as a consequence of crimes committed while mentally unwell. This reflects a complete failure of the approach that argues that patients have a right to choose their care at all times. Gaol is not a place for unwell, mentally ill or drug-dependent patients. Nonetheless, there remains considerable ambivalence over the use of compulsory treatments for mental illness (Callaghan, Ryan & Kerridge, 2013) and variable use of it in practice (Light et al., 2012).

Addiction medicine case presentations

Two case histories are used below to highlight some important clinical and ethical issues in mandatory treatment, involuntary treatment and incarceration that confront both clinicians and dependent individuals.

Case 1

A 35-year-old man, single, has been using multiple drugs in a dependent fashion for 18 years. Family was stable, childhood uneventful. He started drinking alcohol as a 14-year-old schoolboy, escalated to cannabis use and then opioids, and by 19–20 was dependent on benzodiazepines, alcohol and opioids. Treated over the past 15 years with a range of therapies, including,

- residential withdrawal management followed by rehabilitation programs;
- hospital withdrawal management while he received treatment for septic complications of injecting drug use;
- opioid substitution therapy with methadone and buprenorphine; and
- continuous psychosocial support.

When seen in outpatient clinics he is invariably under the influence of benzodiazepines and unable to converse rationally about further management strategies. He contracted the hepatitis C virus through his injecting drug use, and even with the option of the new direct-acting antiviral agents, the patient and his managing clinicians believe that treatment is not appropriate at this time. When he has been incarcerated (on several occasions, for drug-related crimes) his health, both physical and mental, improved dramatically. During incarceration he converses rationally and outlines strategies that might help him stay abstinent in the future. Unfortunately, early release always results in a return to drug use, usually before he makes contact with the health system.

The patient's improvement with abstinence and his willingness to admit he feels better when incarcerated make a case for an involuntary treatment program that would hold him for at least six months to allow a focused treatment program to be implemented to facilitate:

- optimal cerebral function recovery;
- decreased ongoing brain injury;
- stabilisation of the recovery process; and
- establishment of stronger social support systems.

Unfortunately, no data prove this will occur. Notwithstanding this, systemic efforts should be made to demonstrate the capacity of a treatment facility to deliver benefit rather than simply allowing the custodial process to 'take care' of the man's drug problem on an ad hoc basis.

Case 2

A 45-year-old woman with a severe alcohol use disorder has lost her marriage, her work as a secretary, and her self-respect. She is now living in a caravan with a man twice her age who supplies her with alcohol. She returns abnormal liver tests, performs poorly on tests of cognitive function, yet refuses to accept the need for withdrawal management and abstinence as a means of regaining health and minimising further damage. She consumes 100–120 gm (10–12 standard drinks) of alcohol daily. When advised that she could be forced into treatment under the Involuntary Treatment Act of NSW, she decided to accept a referral to a residential rehabilitation program after withdrawal management in the local hospital.

Neither Case 1 nor Case 2 has been forced into treatment against their will. One has demonstrated the value of mandatory abstinence, achieved in prison, and the other demonstrates the power of the capacity to mandate treatment for dependence in driving treatment decisions. Both cases highlight some of the complexities of the patients under consideration in this chapter. Opponents of the concept of mandatory treatment would argue that both these patients are capable of making rational judgements about their drug use and would point to the fact that neither needed mandated care. Case 1, however, will end up in prison again, unless worsening brain injury renders him unable to break the law. Case 2 only accepted treatment when her sole option was involuntary treatment. Her continued refusal of treatment was driven by her desire to drink. In Alcoholics Anonymous terminology, she had not reached 'rock bottom'. But why should a person need to reach total dysfunction and despair before help is provided?

Do drug dependent patients really make rational decisions about their drug use? The following common clinical scenarios suggest that the question is not a simple one. Severely dependent individuals are known to:

- continue drinking despite having experienced two or more life-threatening variceal haemorrhages secondary to alcohol-related cirrhosis. These people are often practising professionals who continue their professional work once they recover from the haemorrhage. The latter strengthens the argument (of opponents to mandatory treatment) that they can indeed make rational choices, but ignores the fact that many professionals can and do continue their professional work despite quite significant cognitive impairment (Cummings, Merlo & Cottler, 2011; Pitkanen, Hurn & Kopelman, 2008);
- continue to inject heroin using shared equipment, despite having lost vision in one eye from fungal ophthalmitis, contracted from contaminated lemon juice used to mix the heroin;
- use amphetamines while practising medicine under the supervision of a State Medical Council. The amphetamine use continues, but is denied, despite thrice-weekly urine drug testing;
- practise as a specialist clinician while denying ongoing use of opioids, despite urine drug screens that identify opioid use; and
- continue to inject benzodiazepines despite losing a limb to vascular damage and gangrene.

These behaviours are hard for healthy rational individuals to comprehend. The dependent individuals often declare their desire to stop behaving in this destructive way, but also declare – equally passionately – that they simply cannot resist the urge to use. A growing body of evidence supports the concept that these individuals are impaired and that their cerebral structure and function are different from those of non-dependent people (Durazzo et al., 2016; Everitt, 2014; Glasser et al., 2016; Hermens et al., 2013; Liao et al., 2016; Narendran et al., 2014; O'Halloran et al., 2017). The jury is still out as to how significant these changes are in determining an individual's capacity to make healthy decisions about ongoing drug use (see Chapter 1, this volume).

Organ damage in drug-using individuals is important to the debate over mandated treatment

Drug use (particularly alcohol use) frequently causes damage to a range of organ systems in the body. Many individuals can use alcohol in large quantities for years without evidence of tissue injury, so researchers must take account of this individual variation in susceptibility to both dependence and organ damage. Drug users vary and we do them a great disservice to assume otherwise.

The central nervous system (CNS) is critical to this discussion, as the brain is the principal organ involved in decision-making processes. Other organs and systems that are vulnerable to damage from dependent drug use include the cardiovascular system, the liver, the pancreas, the peripheral nervous system, the immune system and the lungs (Askgaard et al., 2017; McGaieth & Batey, 2015). Two arguments for compulsory treatment in those who refuse to accept therapy relate to the reality of this organ damage:

- CNS damage occurs much earlier than used to be thought to be the case. New imaging technology demonstrates impaired functional pathways in patients well before overt cognitive impairment is evident. Some studies suggest early damage could be reversible if abstinence can be achieved (Marshall & O'Dell, 2012; Werner & Stevens, 2015). Arguments that patients committed under the Inebriates Act of NSW (1912) showed little response to treatment are meaningless given that these patients had severe and irreversible brain damage from decades of alcohol use. New data continue to document the consequences of drug overdose with hypoxia and hypotension on critical aspects of brain function and anatomy, while expanding our knowledge of the normal brain exponentially (Berrettini, 2016; Durrazo et al., 2016; Glasser et al., 2016).
- Once organ damage exists, ongoing drug use compounds the damage; mandating effective therapy to minimise disease progression makes good public health sense. Askgaard et al. (2017) found an 11-fold increase in cirrhosis risk in men and an 18-fold increase in women admitted to

hospital with alcohol dependence who continue to drink after discharge. The cost to the community of this behaviour is enormous.

Special issues in relation to addiction medicine patients

Drug-dependent individuals often have comorbid mental health diagnoses, but in most patients dependency is the major diagnostic problem (NSW Department of Health, 2009). People with drug dependencies who have minimal or mild mental health pathology present problems that differ from those faced by individuals with a severe mental illness in the following ways:

- they continue to take toxic substances that both impact cerebral function directly and aggravate pre-existing organ damage that further compromises cerebral function via mechanisms such as minimal portal systemic encephalopathy (Patidar & Bajaj, 2015);
- treatments in addiction medicine require a high degree of compliance for prolonged periods and dependent patients find this very hard to achieve; and
- treatments for dependency are only modestly effective in moving individuals to abstinence. If harm reduction is the main goal, treatments can be regarded as modestly effective.

The third point is contentious, but the treatment outcome literature shows that most treatments achieve an abstinence rate at 12 months of far less than 50% for all drugs of dependence studied (Amato et al., 2002; Brensilver, Heinzerling & Shoptaw, 2013; Carson & Taylor, 2014; Del Re et al., 2013; Donoghue et al., 2015; Higuchi et al., 2015; Longo et al., 2010; Mann et al., 2014; Mattick et al., 2009; Mattick et al., 2014; Müller et al., 2014, Pierce et al., 2016; Ponizovsky et al., 2015). Most studies do not even attempt a 12-month follow-up and show less than 50% abstinence rates at only six months of follow-up. Some clinicians argue (from an historical perspective) that a 30% abstinence rate should be accepted as reasonable. This approach to therapy in addiction medicine has held the field back for decades. The fact that outcomes have been poor for 50 years with no improvement in outcomes is as much a reflection on the specialty as it is on the complexity of the disorder. If the same attitude had been held to outcomes for acute leukaemia or hepatitis C we would not now have cures for both conditions (Pui et al., 2014; Shah et al., 2013; Soriano et al., 2016).

The body of literature documenting efficacy for involuntary treatment in addiction medicine is far smaller than that for mental health interventions. A 2005 paper expressed the problems faced by those discussing this topic well: 'Although compulsory/legally mandated treatment is appealing, it has been one of the most fiercely debated topics in the addiction field, raising issues including ethical and motivational considerations' (Klag et al., 2005). Little has changed since 2005, as evidenced by a lack of new studies documenting either the benefit or uselessness of this approach to management. A recent systematic review of research in this arena found only nine of 430 studies met inclusion quality criteria; the conclusion – based largely on only four studies – was that the evidence overall does not suggest improved outcomes related to compulsory treatment approaches (Werb et al., 2016). Given the low success rates of all forms of treatment for drug dependence, any research approach to gaining insight into effective management strategies has to acknowledge that for convincing evidence to be produced, very large cohorts need to be studied. This has not happened to date.

Perhaps the least audited program in the experience of clinicians and individuals in NSW was the original Inebriates Act of 1912, which was used to manage hundreds of individuals over its lifetime. The Act allowed for the mandatory detention of repeatedly inebriated, socially dysfunctional individuals in 'gazetted units' for up to a year. The experience was poor for all concerned (Dore, Batey & Smyth, 2013; Shea, 2005). Despite 100 years of admitting patients under this Act, there was not a single report defining effective management protocols or outcome data. The NSW Inebriates Act was repealed in 2012 and a new Involuntary Treatment Act was passed after detailed discussions between clinicians and policymakers. Two new involuntary treatment units were established in NSW under the new Act: one is in Sydney (four beds) and the other in country NSW (eight beds). A funded review of the two units after four years of operation has not yet been made public. The two units admitted all 303 referred patients between September 2012 and late 2016 (personal communication, NSW Ministry of Health, 2016). This is a far greater number per annum than used to be referred under the Inebriates Act (approximately 10 per year in the final years of the Act). In an interview, a senior staff member of one involuntary treatment unit stated that 'twelve months after discharge one third of the patients are still abstinent and twenty-five per cent on top of that are very significantly improved.' The former figure is quite encouraging, but a published report on the data is awaited eagerly. A publication based on data from the city unit reported that 'while patient numbers are small, treatment responsiveness was evident for 42.5% of patients, most of whom were followed up with assertive community treatment.' The population had high levels of mental health and social comorbidity – mental health comorbidities (97.5%), cortical atrophy (40%) and socioeconomic disadvantage (92.5% were beneficiaries of social supports) (Dore, Sinclair & Murray, 2016).

If these involuntary treatment programs can be shown to deliver better outcomes than current approaches to these highly dependent treatment-resistant patients, mandating more patients could be justified to prevent the development of more severe and potentially irreversible organ damage. Failure to respond to positive data would reflect a dereliction of duty to our patients, who are desperately seeking new options to help them with their life-and-death struggles with dependence.

What involuntary or mandated treatment programs exist for those with a dependency?

In many parts of the world, various forms of involuntary treatment for dependency exist. In Australia, units are being established in several states. They differ from each other in many ways, and the impact of these differences on outcomes should be evaluated. The following section details the various forms of existing programs, focusing on those in Australia. They can be classified according to the structure underpinning them.

Correctional services coerced (involuntary) interventions/treatments

- Pre-sentencing drug diversion options for those facing sentencing because of non-violent, drug related crime. Such programs include the DACAP (Drug and Alcohol Court Assessment Program) and MERIT (Magistrates Early Referral into Treatment) programs in NSW.
- Drug Court programs in which individuals are offered a mandated treatment program instead of a gaol sentence. Failing to adhere to the defined program results in incarceration.

Clinically driven involuntary treatments

- These are involuntary treatments for individuals not involved in crime or not facing an immediate court appearance. They range from restrictions on access to take-away dosing in methadone or buprenorphine programs when rules of the clinic are broken, to more complex protocols designed to improve patient adherence to treatment programs. The conditions surrounding the most restrictive options which include involuntary treatment units vary from state to state, but most insist that all voluntary options have been exhausted, have failed or have been refused by the individual being considered for involuntary treatment. Programs include:

    a   inpatient treatment options; and
    b   outpatient or community-based programs, including community treatment orders.

Mandated treatment strategies for those wishing to continue professional careers while recovering from a dependency problem

- These programs include those that link continuing ability to practise one's profession to engagement in both a treatment program and a monitoring process to demonstrate abstinence from the offending agent(s).

Data exist to suggest each of these specific approaches has value and delivers positive outcomes for at least some of those engaged in them (Clough, Kim San Lee & Conigrave, 2008; Freeman, 2003; Grahn et al., 2015; Nace et al., 2007; Padyab et al., 2015; Pasareanu et al., 2016; Passey, Flaherty & Didcott, 2006; Somers et al., 2012; Vuong et al., 2017; Wild et al., 2016). Despite the theoretical justification that in the absence of data we should not proceed to expand mandatory treatment options (Birgin et al., 2013; Clark, Busse & Gerra, 2013; Hall & Carter, 2013; Macavoy & Flaherty, 1990; see Chapter 1, this volume) these positive reports support the implementation of new research programs to provide data to justify this approach to treatment.

Making a constructive case for a better way forward: a proposal based on the evidence and the lack of it

It is wrong to argue that there are absolutely no data to support the use of involuntary treatments for drug dependency. Some data exist, but unquestionably more are needed. When life-threatening behaviours cannot be ceased because an individual is severely dependent, it is reasonable to suggest a well-designed involuntary treatment program is a less damaging process than allowing the patient to continue uncontrolled drug use. When dependence causes an individual to reject offered treatments, it may be that a period of involuntary treatment is justified. Individual reports from such programs suggest that many patients value their time in involuntary treatment (Dore et al., 2016). The fact that these reports do not have the same strength as a randomised controlled trial is accepted but the results cannot be ignored. On these grounds I argue that mandated treatment for individuals with a severe substance use disorder should be more available. It should be used more frequently under the following conditions.

- Treatments should only be used if all other options have been refused by the individual or have failed because of patient factors. These may include non-completion of the program or adverse consequences from the program. No other, less restrictive options remain.
- The involuntary treatment units are under an obligation to adhere to the following specific requirements:

    a   Full assessment of admitted patients must be undertaken and recorded for evaluation purposes. That assessment process must include a full medical assessment for organ damage known to result from regular drug use, a detailed neuropsychological assessment utilising the latest screening instruments and, where available, neuroimaging performed by teams that are evaluating brain structure/function with relevant resources (such as functional magnetic resonance imaging). It is assumed that detailed history and laboratory-confirmed drug use will be recorded.

b   Data from these units is retained for use in a statewide (preferably nationwide) evaluation of the nature of the patient population and the effects of the interventions on drug use and organ function over a minimum of 12 months from entry to the programs.

c   The services are staffed by professionals with a sound understanding of addiction medicine and a commitment to research designed to progress our understanding of the complexity of dependence.

d   Funding is withdrawn if expected deliverables are not provided on time and consistently.

- Those directing such facilities are chosen because of a proven track record of working collaboratively across the states and territories, as they will need to pool data to allow sample sizes adequate to answer the questions generated at the outset of the process.
- Research expertise is an essential prerequisite of each team; this expertise must include issues of new treatments and the evaluation of the program delivered by the facilities.

If there is to be progress made in understanding dependence through the implementation of these unpopular programs, these involuntary treatment units should be guided by some basic principles:

- current treatments for dependence are relatively ineffective and new data need to drive improvements in therapeutic programs;
- data from new imaging and cognitive testing protocols and from epigenetic studies need to be monitored and incorporated into assessment and treatment programs if they are found to be useful (Berkel & Pandey, 2017);
- dependence at present is poorly understood and continued drug use continues to damage individual users, impairing their capacity to make rational choices about their drug use;
- mandated treatment should only be continued as long as there is evidence that the individual receiving it is not being harmed, is showing evidence of improvement in one or more aspects of their health and well-being, and their experience is being recorded for learning purposes; and
- mandated treatment is not an alternative to incarceration, it is a positive treatment option in its own right.

Conclusion

Despite an absence of convincing data to justify involuntary treatment for dependence, clinical evidence supports the need for a more interventional approach to the care of some severely dependent individuals. These people are notable for the destructive path their drug use is taking, which – if unchecked – will lead to premature death in a significant proportion. I maintain that intervening to provide a period of enforced abstinence is ethically justified, if only to allow adequate time for drug effects to wear off and clearer thought processes to emerge, allowing the individual a better chance to make rational decisions about their subsequent drug use. The fact that we do not have evidence to prove this is worth doing is not so much a scientific deficiency as it is a societal and ethical tragedy.

References

Amato, L., Davoli, M., Ferri, M., & Ali, R. (2002). Methadone at tapered doses for management of opioid withdrawal. *Cochrane Database of Systematic Reviews* 1, CD003409.

Askgaard, G., Leon, D. A., Kjaer, M. S., Deleuran, T., Gerds, T. A., & Tolstrup, J. S. (2017). Risk for alcoholic liver cirrhosis after an inpatient hospital contact with alcohol problems: a nationwide prospective cohort study. *Hepatology* 65(3), 929–937

Bärnighausen, T., Bloom, D. E., Cafiero-Fonseca, E. T., & O'Brien, J. C. (2014). Valuing vaccination. *Proceedings of the National Academy of Sciences of the United States of America* 111, 12313–12319.

Baur, N. (2013). Family influence and psychiatric care: physical treatments in Devon mental hospitals, c. 1920 to the 1970s. *Endeavour*, 37, 172–183.

Bell, J., Trinh, L., Butler, B., Randall, D., & Rubin, G. (2009). Comparing retention in treatment and mortality in people after initial entry to methadone and buprenorphine treatment. *Addiction* 104, 1193–1200.

Berkel, T. D., & Pandey, S. C. (2017). Emerging role of epigenetic mechanisms in alcohol addiction. *Alcoholism, Clinical and Experimental Research*, 41(4), 666–680. doi:10.1111/acer.13338

Berrettini, W. (2016). Opioid neuroscience for addiction medicine: from animal models to FDA approval for alcohol addiction. *Progress in Brain Research* 223, 253–267.

Birgin, R. & Asian Network of People Who Use Drugs (2013). Arguments against the compulsory treatment of opioid dependence. *Bulletin of the World Health Organization* 91, 239–239A.

Brensilver, M., Heinzerling, K. G., & Shoptaw, S. (2013). Pharmacotherapy of amphetamine-type stimulant dependence: an update. *Drug and Alcohol Review* 32(5), 449–460.

Burns, L., Randall, D., Hall, W. D., Law, M., Butler, T., Bell, J., & Degenhardt, L. (2009). Opioid agonist pharmacotherapy in New South Wales from 1985 to 2006: patient characteristics and patterns and predictors of treatment retention. *Addiction* 104, 1363–1372.

Callaghan, S., Ryan, C., & Kerridge, I. (2013). Risk of suicide is insufficient warrant for coercive treatment for mental illness. *International Journal of Law and Psychiatry* 36, 374–385.

Carson, D. S., & Taylor, E. R. (2014). Commentary on Heinzerling et al. (2014): a growing methamphetamine dependence therapeutics graveyard. *Addiction* 109(11), 1887–1888.

Clark, N., Busse, A., & Gerra, G. (2013). Voluntary treatment, not detention, in the management of opioid dependence. *Bulletin of the World Health Organization* 91, 146–147.

Clough, A. R., Kim San Lee, K., & Conigrave, K. M. (2008). Promising performance of a juvenile justice diversion programme in remote Aboriginal communities, Northern Territory, Australia. *Drug and Alcohol Review* 27, 433–438.

Cummings, S. M., Merlo, L., & Cottler, L. (2011). Mechanisms of prescription drug diversion among impaired physicians. *Journal of Addictive Disorders* 30, 195–202.

Del Re, A. C., Maisel, N., Blodgett, J., & Finney, J. (2013). The declining efficacy of naltrexone pharmacotherapy for alcohol use disorders over time: a multivariate meta-analysis. *Alcoholism, Clinical and Experimental Research* 37(6), 1064–1068.

Donoghue, K., Elzerbi, C., Saunders, R., Whittington, C., Pilling, S., & Drummond, C. (2015). The efficacy of acamprosate and naltrexone in the treatment of alcohol dependence, Europe versus the rest of the world: a meta-analysis. *Addiction* 110, 920–930.

Dore, G. M., Batey, R. G., & Smyth, D. J. (2013). Involuntary treatment of drug and alcohol dependence in New South Wales: an old Act and a new direction. *Medical Journal of Australia* 198, 583–585.

Dore, G., Sinclair, B., & Murray, R. (2016). Treatment resistant and resistant to treatment? Evaluation of 40 alcohol dependent patients admitted for involuntary treatment. *Alcohol and Alcoholism* 51, 291–295

Durazzo, T. C., Mon, A., Gazdzinski, S., & Meyerhoff, D. J. (2016). Regional brain volume changes in alcohol-dependent individuals during early abstinence: Associations with relapse following treatment. *Addiction Biology*, June 22. doi:10.1111/adb.12420

Everitt, B. J. (2014). Neural and psychological mechanisms underlying compulsive drug seeking habits and drug memories – indications for novel treatments of addiction. *The European Journal of Neuroscience* 40, 2163–2182.

Freeman, K. (2003). Health and well-being outcomes for drug-dependent offenders on the NSW Drug Court programme. *Drug and Alcohol Review* 22, 409–416.

Galanakis, E., Jansen, A., Lopalco, P. L., & Giesecke, J. (2013). Ethics of mandatory vaccination for healthcare workers. *Euro Surveillance* 18, 20627.

Girotra, S., van Diepen, S., Nallamothu, B. K., Carrel, M., Vellano, K., Anderson, M. L., McNally, B., Abella, B. S., Sasson, C., Chan, P. S., CARES Surveillance Group, & the HeartRescue Project (2016). Regional variation in out-of-hospital cardiac arrest survival in the United States. *Circulation* 133, 2159–2168.

Glasser, M. F., Coalson, T. S., Robinson, E. C., Hacker, C. D., Harwell, J., Yacoub, E., Ugurbil, K., Andersson, J., Beckmann, C. F., Jenkinson, M., Smith, S. M., & Van Essen, D. C. (2016). A multi-modal parcellation of human cerebral cortex. *Nature* 536, 171–178.

Grahn, R., Lundgren, L. M., Chassler, D., & Padyab, M. (2015). Repeated entries to the Swedish addiction compulsory care system: a national register database study. *Evaluation and Program Planning* 49, 163–171.

Halem, S. C. (1997). At what cost? An argument against mandatory AZT treatment of HIV-positive pregnant women. *Harvard Civil Rights–Civil Liberties Law Review* 32, 492–528.

Hall, W., & Carter, A. (2013). Advocates need to show compulsory treatment of opioid dependence is effective, safe and ethical. *Bulletin of the World Health Organization* 91, 146.

Hermens, D. F., Lagopoulos, J., Tobias-Webb, J., De Regt, T., Dore, G., Juckes, L., Latt, N., & Hickie, I. B. (2013). Pathways to alcohol-induced brain impairment in young people: a review. *Cortex* 49, 3–17.

Higuchi, S., & Japanese Acamprosate Study Group (2015). Efficacy of acamprosate for the treatment of alcohol dependence long after recovery from withdrawal syndrome: a randomized, double-blind, placebo-controlled study conducted in Japan (Sunrise Study). *The Journal of Clinical Psychiatry* 76, 181–188.

Klag, S., O'Callaghan, F., & Creed, P. (2005). The use of legal coercion in the treatment of substance abusers: an overview and critical analysis of thirty years of research. *Substance Use & Misuse* 40, 1777–1795.

Laffey, P. (2003). Psychiatric therapy in Georgian Britain. *Psychological Medicine* 33, 1285–1297.

Liao, Y., Tang, J., Liu, J., Xie, A., Yang, M., Johnson, M., Wang, X., Deng, Q., Chen, H., Xiang, X., Liu, T., Chen, X., Song, M., & Hao, W. (2016). Decreased thalamocortical connectivity in chronic ketamine users. *PLoS ONE*, December 15, 11.

Light, E., Kerridge, I., Ryan, C., & Robertson, M. (2012). Community treatment orders in Australia: rates and patterns of use. *Australasian Psychiatry* 20, 478–482.

Longo, M., Wickes, W., Smout, M., Harrison, S., Cahill, S., & White, J. M. (2010). Randomized controlled trial of dexamphetamine maintenance for the treatment of methamphetamine dependence. *Addiction* 105(1), 146–154.

Macavoy, M. G., & Flaherty, B. (1990). Compulsory treatment of alcoholism: the case against. *Drug and Alcohol Review* 9, 267–271.

Mann, K., Vollstädt-Klein, S., Reinhard, I., Leménager, T., Fauth-Bühler, M., Hermann, D., Hoffmann, S., Zimmermann, U.S., Kiefer, F., Heinz, A., & Smolka, M. N. (2014). Predicting naltrexone response in alcohol-dependent patients: the contribution of functional magnetic resonance imaging. *Alcoholism, Clinical and Experimental Research* 38, 2754–2762.

Marshall, J. F., & O'Dell, S. J. (2012). Methamphetamine influences on brain and behavior: unsafe at any speed? *Trends in Neurosciences* 35, 536–545.

Mattick, R. P., Breen, C., Kimber, J., & Davoli, M. (2009). Methadone maintenance therapy versus no opioid replacement therapy for opioid dependence. *Cochrane Database of Systematic Reviews* 2, CD002209.

Mattick, R. P., Breen, C., Kimber, J. & Davoli, M. (2014). Buprenorphine maintenance versus placebo or methadone maintenance for opioid dependence. *Cochrane Database of Systematic Reviews*, 2, CD002207.

McGaieth, S. E., & Batey, R. G. (2015). Liver disorders related to alcohol and other drug use. In A. J. Herron & T. K. Brennan (Eds.), *The ASAM Essentials of Addiction Medicine* (pp. 430–440). Philadelphia: Wolters Kluwer.

Müller, C. A., Geisel, O., Banas, R., & Heinz, A. (2014). Current pharmacological treatment approaches for alcohol dependence. *Expert Opinion on Pharmacotherapy* 15, 471–481.

Nace, E. P., Birkmayer, F., Sullivan, M. A., Galanter, M., Fromson, J. A., Frances, R. J., Levin, F. R., Lewis, C., Suchinsky, R. T., Tamerin, J. S., & Westermeyer, J. (2007). Socially sanctioned coercion mechanisms for addiction treatment. *The American Journal on Addictions* 16, 15–23.

Narendran, R., Mason, N. S., Paris, J., Himes, M. L., Douaihy, A. B., & Frankle, W. G. (2014). Decreased prefrontal cortical dopamine transmission in alcoholism. *The American Journal of Psychiatry* 171, 881–888.

Neugebauer, R. (1979). Medieval and early modern theories of mental health. *Archives of General Psychiatry* 36, 477–483.

NSW Department of Health (Mental Health Branch) (2009). *NSW Clinical Guidelines for the Care of Persons with Comorbid Mental Illness and Substance Use Disorders in Acute Care Settings.* Sydney: NSW Department of Health.

O'Halloran, L., Nymberg, C., Jollans, L., Garavan, H., & Whelan, R. (2017). The potential of neuroimaging for identifying predictors of adolescent alcohol use initiation and misuse. *Addiction* 112, 719–726.

Padyab, M., Grahn, R., & Lundgren, L. (2015). Drop-out from the Swedish addiction compulsory care system. *Evaluation and Program Planning* 49, 178–184.

Pasareanu, A. R., Vederhus, J. K., Opsal, A., Kristensen, O., & Clausen, T. (2016). Improved drug-use patterns at 6 months post-discharge from inpatient substance use disorder treatment: results from compulsorily and voluntarily admitted patients. *BMC Health Services Research* 16, 291–297.

Passey, M., Flaherty, B., & Didcott, P. (2006). The Magistrates Early Referral Into Treatment (MERIT) Pilot Program: a descriptive analysis of a court diversion program in rural Australia. *Journal of Psychoactive Drugs* 38, 521–529.

Patidar, K. R., & Bajaj, J. S. (2015). Covert and overt hepatic encephalopathy: diagnosis and management. *Clinical Gastroenterology and Hepatology* 13, 2048–2061.

Pierce, M., Bird, S. M., Hickman, M., Marsden, J., Dunn, G., Jones, A., & Millar, T. (2016). Impact of treatment for opioid dependence on fatal drug-related poisoning: a national cohort study in England. *Addiction* 111, 298–308.

Pitkanen, M., Hurn, J., & Kopelman, M. D. (2008). Doctors' health and fitness to practise: performance problems in doctors and cognitive impairments. *Occupational Medicine* 58(5), 328–337.

Ponizovsky, A. M., Rosca, P., Aronovich, E., Weizman, A., & Grinshpoon, A. (2015). Baclofen as add-on to standard psychosocial treatment for alcohol dependence: a randomized, double-blind, placebo-controlled trial with 1 year follow-up. *Journal of Substance Abuse Treatment* 52, 24 30.

Pui, H., Pei, D., Campana, D., Cheng, C., Sandlund, J. T., Bowman, W. P., Hudson, M. M., Ribeiro, R. C., Raimondi, S. C., Jeha, S., Howard, S. C., Bhojwani, D., Inabam, H., Rubnitz, J. E., Metzger, M. L., Gruber, T. A., Coustan-Smith, E., Downing, J. R., Leung, W. H., Relling, M. V., & Evans, W. E. (2014). A revised definition for cure of childhood acute lymphoblastic leukemia. *Leukemia* 28(12), 2336–2343.

Randall, L. H., Curran, E. A., & Omer, S.B. (2013). Legal considerations surrounding mandatory influenza vaccination for healthcare workers in the United States. *Vaccine* 31, 1771–1776.

Shah, A., Andersson, T. M., Rachet, B., Björkholm, M., & Lambert, P.C. (2013). Survival and cure of acute myeloid leukaemia in England, 1971–2006: a population-based study. *British Journal of Haematology* 162(4), 509–516.

Shea, P. (2005). The New South Wales Inebriates Act: going, going, gone? *Australasian Psychiatry* 13, 195–197.

Somers, J. M., Currie, L., Moniruzzaman, A., Eiboff, F., & Patterson, M. (2012). Drug treatment court of Vancouver: an empirical evaluation of recidivism. *International Journal of Drug Policy* 23, 393–400.

Soriano, V., Labarga, P., Fernandez-Montero, J. V., de Mendoza, C., Esposito, I., Benítez-Gutiérrez, L., & Barreiro, P. (2016). Hepatitis C cure with antiviral therapy – benefits beyond the liver. *Antiviral Therapy* 21(1), 1–8.

Vuong, T., Nguyen, N., Giang, L., Shanahan, M., Ali, R., & Ritter, A. (2017). The political and scientific challenges in evaluating compulsory drug treatment centres in Southeast Asia. *Harm Reduction Journal* 14, 2–16.

Werb, D., Kamarulzaman, A., Meacham, M. C., Rafful, C., Fischer, B., Strathdee, S. A., & Wood, E. (2016). The effectiveness of compulsory drug treatment: a systematic review. *International Journal of Drug Policy* 28, 1–9.

Werner, J. K., & Stevens, R. D. (2015). Traumatic brain injury: recent advances in plasticity and regeneration. *Current Opinion in Neurology* 28, 565–573.

Wild, T. C., Yuan, Y., Rush, B. R., & Urbanoski, K. A. (2016). Client engagement in legally-mandated addiction treatment: a prospective study using self-determination theory. *Journal of Substance Abuse Treatment* 69, 35–43.

Wu, Z. (2013). Arguments in favour of compulsory treatment of opioid dependence. *Bulletin of the World Health Organization* 91, 142–145.

Part II

Lives, bodies and voices - The material impacts and lived effects of coercion

In the first part of this book, we considered some of the arguments for and against the use of coercive treatment. Those contributions focused primarily on claims about the ethics of coerced forms of treatment, and debates about whether these practices are supported by evidence.

In this part, we examine a very different set of questions about the appropriateness of coercive practices. Focusing on the lives, bodies and voices of those most closely affected, we explore the material impacts and lived effects of coercion. We ask: is coercive treatment just? Is coercive treatment always already unjust? Is it a form of unjust and unjustifiable violence? We also ask: who speaks and who can speak about the lived experience of such treatment? Is it ever possible to know coercive treatment from the perspective of those most directly affected, and if not, what are the implications of this?

This part features contributions from three very different perspectives. The first is from Australian lawyer Eleanore Fritze, who writes about her experience of representing people subjected to coercive treatment (with a focus on people thought to be experiencing mental health problems). The second piece is by consumer academic Cath Roper. She writes about her own experiences as a patient subjected to coerced mental health treatment, and explores the attempted justifications for the treatment administered to her. Finally, Claire Spivakovsky examines attempts to give voice and/or bear witness to the violence and abuse perpetrated upon people living with disability, and the impossibility of ever adequately doing so.

Although Fritze, Roper and Spivakovsky come from different perspectives, are concerned with the experiences of different populations and examine these practices from different positions and perspectives, two common themes emerge. The first involves the paramount importance of assessing claims about the value of coercive treatment from the perspective of those who are most directly affected by it. The second involves the need to consider questions of justice and injustice when discussing the merits, effects and effectiveness of coerced treatment. This second point requires some further explanation.

Questions about justice (and injustice) are central to a range of fields, including law, criminology and philosophy. In recent years, Miranda Fricker's (2007) work on epistemic injustice has urged us to think about justice and injustice in new ways, by focusing not simply on the outcome of formal legal proceedings but on what happens along the way. Fricker argues that practices may be unjust when they impact on the capacity of subjects to know and to be known. This is a distinct form of injustice that requires consideration quite separately from assessments of the formal outcomes, for instance, of legal proceedings. Explaining the concept of epistemic injustice as a discrete but common form of injustice, Fricker explains that:

> any epistemic injustice wrongs someone in their capacity as a subject of knowledge, and thus in a capacity essential to human value; and the particular way in which testimonial injustice does this is that a hearer wrongs a speaker in his [sic] capacity as a giver of knowledge, as an informant. I argue that the primary harm one incurs in being wronged in this way is an intrinsic injustice.
>
> (2007, p. 5)

Applying these insights to her own experiences with coercive treatment, Cath Roper argues that coercive treatment reduces one's capacity as a knower. In this sense, coercive treatment is arguably always already unjust. One reason for this is that coercive treatment is frequently underpinned by or involves doubt about the reliability and credibility of those who are labelled 'mentally ill'. Coercive treatment and the practices that enable it often foreclose opportunities to hear from those who are affected, or to allow them to speak as valid, credible subjects.

Eleanore Fritze approaches the question of experience, voice, absence and silence from an altogether different perspective: that of the lawyer seeking to advocate for and give voice to those who have experienced or are at risk of experiencing some form of coercive treatment. Recounting tales from the frontline, on behalf of herself and her colleagues, Fritze outlines the tendency in legal processes to silence and obscure the voices of those so affected. Legal practices are thus frequently unjust, through their capacity to both reproduce the epistemic forms of injustice highlighted by Fricker, and through the denial of basic rights – including a thorough testing of the evidence supporting coercive treatment – especially for clients who do not have legal representation.

Claire Spivakovsky's work also speaks to epistemic injustice, within the context of disability settings. Arguing that personal accounts of coercive interventions (or 'restrictive practices') are painfully absent from the public discourse, she examines whether, how and why it is possible for people with disability to give voice to their experiences of ill-treatment, violence and abuse. She argues that people with disability who experience certain kinds of coercive interventions are denied the common vocabulary to voice the violence of coercive interventions, and outlines some of the ways in which their accounts become simultaneously impossible or counterproductive. She argues that even when formal processes (such as parliamentary committees) seek to give voice to those affected by these practices, they may paradoxically work to stabilise the conditions and logics of violence and abuse, instantiating a fundamentally flawed and unjust ableist narrative.

The contributions in this part encourage us to confront some uncomfortable questions about coercive treatment and the power of the law. Together, they speak not only to the idea that coercive treatment is a form of unjustifiable violence, but to the notion that the material–discursive practices that enable coercive treatment are themselves hugely problematic, unethical, and often unjust. These insights raise profound and disturbing questions about how we treat some of society's most vulnerable citizens and the harms that might be perpetrated upon them in the name of justice. If coercive treatment is inherently unjust, can it ever be warranted?

Chapter 4

The variable treatment of (in)capacity in the practical operation of Victoria's key substituted decision-making regimes

View from the frontline

Eleanore Fritze[1]

Various laws in Victoria, including the *Mental Health Act 2014* (MHA), *Guardianship and Administration Act 1986* (GAA), *Disability Act 2006* and *Severe Substance Dependence Treatment Act 2010*, permit people with mental illness, disabilities and/or substance dependence to be detained, subjected to compulsory treatment and deprived of their decision-making rights in a range of ways. The curtailment of people's autonomy and freedoms under these laws is typically, although not always explicitly, justified in the name of incapacity. Each regime, however, gives differing relevance to, and posits different tests and thresholds for, (in)capacity. This chapter examines how the concept of capacity is treated under the two Acts which affect by far the greatest number of people: the GAA and the MHA. In doing so, it looks beyond what the laws say on their face about (in)capacity to how they are interpreted and applied in practice, and explores some of the common assumptions that decision-makers appear to use to justify their decisions to restrict a person's autonomy. The examination reveals generally limited explicit consideration or exploration of decision-making capacity, a tendency to defer to clinical opinion and an orientation towards outcomes, wellbeing and protectionist concerns beyond the strict parameters of the Acts. This raises questions about the proper scope of the tribunals' role and the justifiability of their interventions.

This chapter draws on the collective experience of lawyers (including the author) in Victoria Legal Aid's (VLA)[2] Mental Health and Disability Law (MHDL) program, distilled from our case data, intra-office discussions over many years, and an online survey.[3] VLA is Victoria's largest provider of legal services in relation to these laws. In 2015–2016, we collectively appeared in over 1100 Mental Health Tribunal (MHT) hearings and over 120 GAA hearings at the Victorian Civil and Administrative Tribunal (VCAT), in each case acting on behalf (and on the instructions) of the person with the (alleged) mental illness or disability. Because of our role, we are in a unique position to observe these decision-makers in action.

There are clearly limitations in drawing on lawyers' experiences as a source of information about decision-makers' assumptions and approaches to (in)capacity. We do not appear in every hearing[4] and, when we do, decision-makers may act and speak differently, such that the hearings we experience are not necessarily typical of all hearings. There is also an inherent subjectivity in this approach because it relies to a degree on inferences being drawn from decision-makers' lines of questioning, comments, tone or demeanour during a hearing. Furthermore, there is likely to be a degree of bias, even if unconscious, in lawyers evaluating hearings in which they were active participants on behalf of one party, especially given our strong rights focus and inclination towards the rule of law. However, despite these limitations, this information is not readily obtainable from other sources. No others observe such a broad range of decision-makers within and across these jurisdictions, especially as MHT hearings are closed to the public (MHA s 193). Written statements of reasons or judgments are only occasionally produced[5] and, even if they are, they are not necessarily a complete,[6] accurate or neutral record of the hearing or the reasons and motives underpinning the decision (Peay, 1989, p. 216). Accordingly, the perspectives and information of lawyers who frequently appear in these jurisdictions makes a unique and valuable contribution to understanding how (in)capacity is dealt with in practice.

The Guardianship and Administration Act

The GAA permits the appointment of guardians and administrators to make substituted decisions about various matters on behalf of persons with a 'disability' (defined to mean 'intellectual impairment, mental disorder, brain injury, physical disability or dementia' – GAA s 3(1)). The concept of incapacity is directly incorporated into the second criterion for making an order: the person must be 'unable by reason of the disability to make reasonable judgments in respect of all or any of the matters relating to [their] person or circumstances' (GAA s 22(1)(b)) (in the case of a guardianship order) or in respect of 'all or any part of [their] estate' (GAA s 46(1)(a)(ii)) (in the case of an administration order). The remaining criteria are that the person 'needs' a substituted decision-maker (GAA ss 22(1)(c), 46(1)(a)(iii)) and that making the order would be in their 'best interests' (GAA ss 22(3), 46(3)).

If the incapacity criterion is strictly applied, orders cannot be made where the person is *able* to make (objectively) reasonable judgments but chooses not to. Rather than simply examining the decisions which the person has made or intends to make, the criterion requires a focus on the decision-making process itself. It is thus more respectful of autonomy and the 'dignity of risk' (the right, and importance for self-determination of being able, to make decisions that involve a degree of risk and with which others may disagree) compared to other substituted decision-making regimes such as the MHA and *Disability Act 2006*, which permit decisions made with capacity to be overridden. It is also clear from the criterion's wording that the person's capacity should be assessed in relation to their particular circumstances rather than against some objective standard or the routine affairs of an 'ordinary' person. Thus, a person with complex financial affairs, for instance involving business assets or a large inheritance, will need a commensurately higher level of decision-making ability to manage those affairs and preserve their autonomy than a person with simple affairs. This means that the threshold for capacity is fluid, reflecting the well-accepted principle that capacity is decision- and context-specific.

Parliament, through the inclusion of section 4(2), requires the GAA to be interpreted, and every function, power and discretion exercised or performed, so that:

- the means which are least restrictive of a person's freedom of decision and action are adopted;
- the best interests of the person with a disability are promoted; and
- the person's wishes are given effect to wherever possible.

However, the GAA provides no detail or practical guidance on *how* VCAT should determine whether a person is 'unable to make reasonable judgments'.

VCAT's application of the incapacity criterion

In the experience of MHDL lawyers, VCAT typically insists on clinical evidence regarding a person's capacity prior to listing a hearing, and frequently defers to such evidence in making its decision. Although it is an error of law for VCAT to treat an expert opinion as conclusive of an issue, thereby abdicating its role as decision-maker (*XYZ v State Trustees Ltd* (2006) 25 VAR 402, pp. 423–424), almost all MHDL lawyers surveyed reported that VCAT 'hardly ever' or only 'sometimes' conducts its own assessment during the hearing of the person's ability to make reasonable decisions. This suggests that VCAT members tend to see the ability to make reasonable decisions as a clinical rather than legal question.

In our experience, VCAT sets a low threshold for the evidence it requires to make a GAA order. When hearing an initial application, the evidence before VCAT regarding incapacity is typically a box ticked on a template medical report form that states, 'The person is unable to make reasonable decisions'. The information recorded in the space below as to how this opinion was formed is rarely detailed or referrable to decision-making processes (for example, 'Still unwell'), and is sometimes blank. Furthermore, the person who completed the form rarely attends the hearing, making it difficult to explore or challenge the basis on which the box was ticked. However, orders are frequently made on such evidence.

When considering GAA applications, VCAT gives strong weight to considerations of the person's 'best interests', sometimes to such a degree that they appear to obscure consideration of whether the primary criteria are actually met. VCAT sometimes also incorrectly (*XYZ v State Trustees Ltd* (2006) 25 VAR 402, p. 420; *Patrick's Case* (2011) 39 VR 373, p. 381) conflates the distinct questions of 'incapacity' and 'need' for a substituted decision-maker. For instance, in considering how VCAT approaches the incapacity criterion, almost all MHDL lawyers surveyed 'somewhat' or 'strongly' agreed that VCAT members appear to:

- consider decisions which are not in a person's objective best interests as evidence of the person's inability to make reasonable decisions;
- apply different standards for different classes of people based on their perceived vulnerability (such as old or young age, or being in hospital);
- make and confirm orders to manage behaviours considered problematic (such as drug-taking or gambling); and
- make and confirm orders to protect the person from others who are likely to manipulate or take advantage of them (such as a family member spending their pension for their own purposes).

This last category is particularly concerning because it involves significant restrictions (i.e., orders) being placed on the autonomy and privacy of persons with disability to protect them from improper and sometimes criminal behaviour of others, rather than because they themselves are unable to make decisions (the latter consideration often being glossed over in favour of protectionism).

To properly assess a person's capacity, it is necessary to understand their explanations and motivations for making decisions or permitting circumstances which may otherwise appear contrary to their objective best interests. As Simon's case below demonstrates, this requires engaging directly with the person. However, we understand that most GAA hearings proceed in the person's absence. The Victorian Law Reform Commission (VLRC) reported that VCAT does not collect data on attendance at GAA hearings but noted that it 'does not occur in many cases' (VLRC, 2012, p. 470). Non-attendance seriously limits VCAT's ability to properly explore and determine the person's decision-making capacity.

Box 4.1 Simon's case[7]

Simon had been detained in a psychiatric hospital for decades and had accumulated considerable savings (which he held in a regular bank account rather than a higher-interest facility). However, he refused to regularly purchase new clothes for himself, despite some having holes or stains or being ill-fitting. Concerned about these and other matters, the hospital applied for an administration order over him. At the hearing, Simon articulated the reasoning behind each of his decisions. For instance, he refused to regularly purchase new clothes because, in his opinion, his existing clothes were adequately warm and functional and, consistent with his long-held values, he did not want to waste resources. He also felt that his personal presentation was one of the few means he had left to express his individuality, given the other constraints on his freedom. He resisted pressure to invest his money because he wanted to keep his finances simple: he was familiar with the processes required to access his funds and enjoyed knowing the full amount was available to him whenever he might want it, and he did not want to have to learn any new process or account details at his advanced age. After hearing Simon's explanations and submissions from his lawyer, VCAT dismissed the application because it could not be satisfied that he was unable to make reasonable decisions about his financial affairs. In doing so, the VCAT member emphasised the dignity of risk and the role of personal values in decision-making.

Despite a requirement that any administration order made is 'the least restrictive of that person's freedom of decision and action as is possible in the circumstances' (GAA s 46(4)), VCAT typically defaults to making plenary administration orders, which give the administrator control over the person's entire estate, and rather than limiting the order to the specific matters about which there is evidence the person is unable to make reasonable decisions. The VLRC (2012, p. 26) reported that limited administration orders are 'rare', with only 12 out of 9000 orders appointing State Trustees[8] as administrator in 2008–2009 being limited. However, while the scope of restrictions imposed on people's autonomy and privacy with respect to their financial affairs is often greater than demonstrated to be necessary, VCAT takes a different approach with guardianship orders. Guardianship orders are typically limited to the specific health and lifestyle decisions which need to be made in the foreseeable future and which the person has been found to be unable to decide themselves, and plenary guardianship orders are 'rare' (VLRC, 2012, p. 26). This difference in approach is likely to be because:

- many guardianship applications relate to a specific, discrete issue that needs to be decided (such as where the person should live) rather than regular or recurring decisions (such as paying bills);
- the Office of the Public Advocate (OPA),[9] which typically adopts a considered, rights-respecting position, is regularly involved in guardianship matters (either as a party or following a request by VCAT to investigate and report on a matter pursuant to *Victorian Civil and Administrative Tribunal Act 1998* (Vic) sch 1 cl 45), but is much less frequently involved in administration order matters; and

- there is perhaps a perception that it is less invasive or distressing to have another person make financial decisions than seemingly more personal health and lifestyle decisions.

Duration and review of GAA orders

Although the orders last indefinitely, VCAT is required to conduct periodic 'reassessments' (GAA s 61(1)), which are usually done every 12 months for guardianship orders and three years for administration orders (VLRC, 2012, p. 471). In the experience of MHDL lawyers, VCAT defaults to this three-year timeframe regardless of whether there is evidence to suggest that the criteria will remain met throughout that time. This is problematic because VCAT's orders are made following a snapshot, point-in-time assessment of the person and their circumstances, yet the restrictions on their rights and freedoms remain in place for years to come. Again, the difference in approach likely reflects the more confined scope of guardianship orders and OPA's involvement.

At law, each reassessment hearing requires a fresh examination of the evidence against the criteria; the existing order is not to be regarded as presumptively correct even if the evidence before VCAT is unchanged (*McDonald v Guardianship and Administration Board* [1993] 1 VR 521, pp. 533–534). However, most MHDL lawyers surveyed perceived that VCAT operates under an assumption that, once there is evidence a person lacks decision-making capacity, the person continues to lack capacity until there is new evidence that proves they *do* have capacity. Our practice experience, exemplified by Samir's case below, is that VCAT will typically keep confirming administration orders upon reassessment, even in the absence of current or cogent evidence, until presented with evidence positively disproving the criteria and/or until a lawyer challenges them about the absence of evidence. VCAT's practice of requiring fresh evidence positively disproving the criteria is also reflected in a recently-produced guide for administrators, which states 'VCAT will need medical or psychological reports, or both, to support revoking the administration order' (OPA and State Trustees, 2017, p. 31). Orders are also sometimes confirmed despite the person providing VCAT with positive, recent evidence that their condition is well under control and not interfering with their decision-making ability, as in Marguerita's case below. This approach not only reverses the tests under the GAA, it conflicts with the well-accepted principle that capacity can and does vary over time, particularly where the person has an episodic or fluctuating condition like mental illness.

Box 4.2 Samir's case

Samir was placed on an administration order in the context of schizophrenia, heroin use and homelessness. The order was confirmed upon reassessment on eight separate occasions over the next 16 years. Throughout this time, the only evidence on VCAT's file which addressed his decision-making ability remained one sentence written by his then-case manager in the initial application: he 'hasn't lived independently previously, has poor coping/problem solving skills, behaves impulsively, has minimal insight into difficulties he has with day-to-day living.' However, Samir had since commenced treatment with clozapine, which had been largely effective in stabilising his illness, and was living in a controlled, drug-free environment. The order, which had been in place for 18 years, was revoked after Samir engaged a lawyer.

Marguerita's case

Marguerita was placed on an administration order during a hospital admission for her mental illness. Over 20 years later, the order remained in place. Marguerita had provided VCAT with reports from her doctor over several years, which positively stated she *was* able to make reasonable decisions. However, VCAT confirmed the order upon reassessment at least twice more. Marguerita then engaged a lawyer and the order was revoked.

VCAT requires people to 'opt in' to their periodic reassessment hearings; unless they do, VCAT will conduct the reassessment 'on the papers' (without an actual hearing). Consequently, most reassessments occur in the absence of the person or any current evidence, making a proper assessment of the person's (in)capacity at that time practically impossible. As the above case examples demonstrate, the level of scrutiny which VCAT appears to apply when conducting reassessments on the papers is inconsistent and sometimes questionable. Tim's case below is a particularly concerning example.

Box 4.3 Tim's case

A lawyer represented Tim in his application to revoke his administration order. At the conclusion of the hearing, the VCAT member reserved her judgment. She later recorded her decision in the physical file that the order should be revoked because the criteria were not met. However, due to an administrative error, her decision was not entered in VCAT's system or conveyed to the parties. Subsequently, the matter came on for periodic reassessment. Without any notice of hearing being sent to Tim or his lawyer, a different VCAT member proceeded to conduct a reassessment on the papers and confirmed the order, seemingly without having opened the file to see the recent hearing notes and decision to revoke by the first member.

It is notable that guardianship orders do not linger in place in the way that administration orders do. This is evident from the breakdown between initial and reassessment hearings for the different types of orders. For instance, in 2014–2015, 83% (6442) of all administration order hearings were reassessments of existing orders rather than initial applications, whereas only 27% (783) of guardianship order hearings were reassessments (VCAT, 2015, p. 33). The difference in these figures is more striking when it is remembered that VCAT defaults to spacing out reassessments of administration orders at three-yearly rather than annual intervals. State Trustees reported that the average length of orders appointing them as administrator, including those currently in force, was 6.72 years (VLRC, 2012, p. 471). However, MHDL lawyers frequently encounter orders that have been in place for decades.

Over the last few years, MHDL lawyers have made concerted efforts to advocate against administration orders being made or confirmed in the absence of current or cogent evidence establishing the criteria are met in every case in which our assistance is sought. Half of MHDL lawyers surveyed either 'somewhat' or 'strongly' felt that VCAT had become better at correctly applying the law (including evidentiary burdens) over the last five years (with the other half feeling neutral or that it was still too variable to say). Most lawyers also 'somewhat' agreed with the proposition that, when a lawyer (rather than the person alone) appears at a hearing and challenges the absence of current or cogent evidence, the VCAT member will now usually accept that they cannot confirm the order. However, as the rate of legal representation in these matters is very low,[10] it is unclear whether this shift is also occurring in the majority of cases in which the person represents themselves or does not attend.

In the experience of MHDL lawyers, as VCAT increasingly accepts that it cannot make or confirm orders in the absence of cogent evidence satisfying the criteria, it has become more likely to delay finalisation and/or take steps to obtain new evidence before revoking an order or dismissing an application. Where there is a clear basis for concern, it may be appropriate for VCAT, as an inquisitorial decision-making body, to refer a matter to OPA for investigation. However, in some cases – such as Max's below – there does not seem to be a clear justification for delaying finalisation, especially when the matter is adjourned without any steps being taken to obtain new information. This apparent reluctance to 'let go' suggests that, rather than approaching cases from a neutral, detached position, some VCAT members feel quite protective and invested in the person's future, which raises questions about the proper scope of VCAT's role.

Box 4.4 Max's case

Vincent applied to VCAT for a guardianship and administration order in respect of his son, Max, who has a mental illness. The only medical evidence in support of Vincent's application was a letter from Vincent's own psychologist, who said he had seen Max once several years ago and speculated about the nature of his condition. At the first hearing, the matter was adjourned to obtain more information about Max's financial affairs. At the second hearing, VCAT adjourned the matter to seek a medical report from Max's current treating team. This report, provided prior to the third hearing, positively stated that Max could make reasonable decisions. However, rather than dismiss the application, VCAT adjourned the matter with a request that OPA conduct an investigation. At the next hearing, VCAT adjourned the case again with a direction that Max provide a written statement setting out his proposals for managing his financial affairs. Max provided the statement as directed and asked VCAT to dismiss the application. However, VCAT then ordered Max to provide a copy of any legal or other advice he had received regarding his financial affairs. Max declined to provide this on the basis that it was subject to legal professional privilege, and again asked VCAT to dismiss the application for lack of evidence. VCAT set the matter down for yet another hearing. On this occasion, a different VCAT member conducted the hearing and dismissed the application, over 50 weeks after it was first made.

The Mental Health Act

The other major substituted decision-making regime in Victoria is the MHA, which permits compulsory treatment for mental illness pursuant to a treatment order where the 'treatment criteria' in section 5 are satisfied. These are that:

- the person has 'mental illness' (defined as 'a medical condition … characterised by a significant disturbance of thought, mood, perception or memory', subject to certain qualifications – MHA s 4);
- because of that illness, immediate treatment is necessary to prevent 'serious deterioration' in the person's mental or physical health or 'serious harm' to themselves or others;
- the treatment will be provided to the person if they are subject to a treatment order; and
- 'there is no less restrictive means reasonably available to enable the person to receive the immediate treatment.'

This final, 'least restrictive' criterion requires the decision-maker (the authorised psychiatrist, in relation to temporary treatment orders, or the MHT, in relation to longer-term orders) to consider whether adequate treatment can be received voluntarily, in the absence of an order compelling the person to accept it. By default, a treatment order authorises compulsory treatment in the community but, if the decision-maker is satisfied that treatment 'cannot occur within the community', they can make an inpatient treatment order (ITO) which authorises detention and treatment in a designated mental health service (MHA ss 45, 48(3), 52, 55(3)).

Relevance of (in)capacity under the MHA

Prior to July 2014, under the *Mental Health Act 1986* (Vic) (MHA 1986), it was an additional criterion for compulsory treatment that the person 'ha[d] refused or [was] unable to consent to the necessary treatment for the mental illness' (MHA 1986, s 8(1)(d)). This two-pronged criterion meant that:

- people who had capacity to make an informed refusal of treatment could still be subjected to compulsory treatment; and
- any acquiescence or expressed willingness to comply with treatment had to be scrutinised to determine whether it constituted informed consent, which was often a demeaning and disempowering process in practice and commonly resulted in the person being found to lack capacity.

However, this criterion was not replicated in MHA 2014, which allows a willingness to accept treatment to defeat the least restrictive criterion and prevent a treatment order being made without having to scrutinise whether that willingness is underpinned by informed consent. While it is almost certainly contrary to international human rights law that the MHA still permits compulsory treatment of persons with capacity to make their own treatment decisions (e.g. Callaghan & Ryan, 2016, p. 610), the removal of the requirement to demonstrate capacity where a person is accepting treatment is at least consistent with the person-centred and rights-focused principles underpinning the reforms (e.g. MHA ss 11(1)(a), 11(1)(d), 70(2), set out below), as it implicitly reflects a presumption that the person has capacity and affords more people the dignity of being treated voluntarily.

In applying the least restrictive criterion, the MHT rarely expressly considers whether a person's willingness to comply with treatment is an informed decision made with capacity; more than half of MHDL lawyers reported they had never seen the MHT actively consider the person's capacity to give informed consent to treatment during a treatment order hearing. There does not appear to be a concern that people with mental illness who lack capacity to give informed consent will be disadvantaged or subject to overbearing pressure by services if no treatment order is made to formally authorise – and permit external scrutiny of – the treatment to which they are acquiescing. This contrasts with VCAT's approach to compulsory treatment for people with intellectual disabilities under the *Disability Act 2006*.[11]

While the MHT is not required to consider a person's capacity in treatment order hearings, the MHA requires authorised psychiatrists to consider it in relation to each specific, proposed treatment. Before any treatment is administered to a person, even someone subject to a treatment order, the MHA requires that their informed consent is sought (MHA s 70(1)), and the person seeking their consent must presume they have capacity to give it (MHA s 70(2)). A person 'has the capacity to give informed consent' if they understand the information given to them that is relevant to the decision, are able to remember and use or weigh that information, and are able to communicate their decision in some way (MHA s 68(1)). The MHA sets out some principles to guide this assessment, including that capacity is decision-specific and may change over time, incapacity cannot be assumed based on appearance or other characteristics or based only on the person making a decision that could be considered unwise, and reasonable steps should be taken to conduct the assessment at a time when and in an environment where the person's capacity can be assessed most accurately (MHA s 68(2)). If the person is unable or refuses to provide informed consent to the proposed treatment, the authorised psychiatrist may only make a compulsory treatment decision (giving substituted consent for a particular treatment, other than electroconvulsive treatment or neurosurgery for mental illness) if satisfied that there is no less restrictive way to treat the person (MHA s 71(1), (3)).

This dialogue about proposed treatments and treatment preferences, and any examination of whether the presumption of capacity has been displaced, ought to occur prior to the authorised psychiatrist forming an opinion that compulsory treatment is required, well before the matter ever comes before the MHT. However, how these provisions are applied in practice remains unclear because, in the experience of MHDL lawyers, these discussions and decisions are generally poorly documented in patient files. Furthermore, despite the central relevance of particular treatment decisions in determining whether compulsory treatment is required (particularly as many people are willing to accept some treatment, even if not the psychiatrist's preferred treatment), it is the experience of MHDL lawyers that many MHT members are reluctant to examine or comment on specific treatment decisions in the course of treatment order hearings, despite the MHT's own guidance materials acknowledging that it may be helpful to do so from a 'solution-focused' perspective (MHT, 2014, p. 21). Further research is required to explore whether and how psychiatrists apply these compulsory treatment decision-making provisions in practice.

MHT's application of the least restrictive criterion

In deciding whether the treatment criteria apply, the MHT must have regard to various factors 'to the extent that is reasonable in the circumstances', including 'the person's views and preferences about treatment of [their] mental illness and the reasons for those views and preferences, including any recovery outcomes that the person would like to achieve' (MHA s 55(2)(a)). The MHT must also have regard to the 'mental health principles', which include that persons receiving mental health services should:

- be 'provided assessment and treatment in the least restrictive way possible with voluntary assessment and treatment preferred';
- be 'provided those services with the aim of bringing about the best possible therapeutic outcomes and promoting recovery and full participation in community life';
- be 'involved in all decisions about their assessment, treatment and recovery and be supported to make, or participate in, those decisions, and their views and preferences should be respected';
- be 'allowed to make decisions about their assessment, treatment and recovery that involve a degree of risk'; and
- have 'their rights, dignity and autonomy respected and promoted' (MHA s 11(1)(a)-(e)).

In the majority of MHT cases in which MHDL lawyers appear, the person expresses a willingness and intention to comply with at least adequate or minimally necessary treatment and thus it is argued on their behalf that the least restrictive criterion is not met. However, while dissatisfaction of the least restrictive criterion is the most frequent basis on which the MHT revokes treatment orders (MHT, 2016, p. 18), the MHT does not simply accept stated intentions to comply at face value: MHDL lawyers reported that this argument is accepted in less than a quarter of cases in which it is run, with the MHT deciding that compulsory treatment is necessary in the remaining cases.

Rather than incapacity, the MHT's focus under the least restrictive criterion seems to be on the practical likelihood of voluntary compliance. The MHT regularly appears to conclude that the person will not put into effect or sustain their stated intention to comply because of continuing active symptoms, a limited understanding about their illness and treatment ('lack of insight') and/or lifestyle factors (such as substance use or homelessness). Provided there is evidence to support it, such scenarios may justify a finding that there is no less restrictive way of ensuring the treatment is received than by making a treatment order. However, in the experience of most MHDL lawyers, there does not seem to be a cogent evidentiary basis in half or more of these cases for the MHT to disregard the person's stated intention to comply with treatment and find the criterion satisfied at that particular time.

One common but flawed[12] approach that some MHT members adopt is to justify their satisfaction of the least restrictive criterion by the severity of the harms or consequences that are present or might eventuate should non-compliance or relapse occur (i.e., the strength with which the second criterion is met), regardless of the person's current mental state or any reason to doubt their likelihood of compliance. This concern to avoid negative consequences, which is reminiscent of the 'best interests' considerations under the GAA, is evident in the following justifications, which most MHDL lawyers reported hearing frequently when their client's stated intention to comply with treatment is rejected:

- 'you were very unwell when you came into hospital/recently';
- 'we just want to make sure you get the treatment'; and
- 'we just want to give you the best chance of recovery'.

In other cases, the MHT appears to rely on previous non-compliance to find the least restrictive criterion satisfied, regardless of the passage of time since that non-compliance and/or any changes in the person's circumstances that might significantly improve the likelihood of future compliance. If positive intentions to comply have started being expressed only recently, the MHT will often be reticent to accept them, even when it is the person's first experience of mental ill-health (and so quite understandable that they had been hesitant about accepting treatment prior to psychoeducation and/or the reduction of symptoms). The MHT is meant to assess whether the treatment criteria apply – and thus whether compulsory treatment is required – at that particular point in time. Basing decisions on a person's past statements or behaviour risks failing to acknowledge the progress they have made, which people frequently find discouraging and frustrating. It is also potentially a missed opportunity to capitalise on their current engagement and afford them the dignity of voluntary treatment.

As with GAA orders, MHDL lawyers reported that it was common for the MHT to apply different standards for different classes of people based on their perceived vulnerability or the consequences at stake for them if they relapsed or became non-compliant in the future. For example, in one hearing, a lawyer representing a 16-year-old made submissions about the narrow definition of a particular term in the MHA, which did not apply to the person's circumstances. The psychiatrist MHT member interrupted the lawyer to say pointedly, 'we are talking about a child'. The MHT, by majority, went on to reject the legal submission and made a treatment order because, they said, they were 'bound by the principle of fair-mindedness'; the legal member dissented. Other cohorts besides children that appear to attract shifting standards include young women (particularly those who are sexually active, seen as sexually vulnerable, or pregnant), mothers of infants and young children and those whose reputation, career or potential may suffer if clinical recovery, and behaviour seen as appropriate, are not assured through continued compulsory treatment.

Finally, one of the most frequent expressions which MHDL lawyers reported hearing from the MHT when a treatment order is made, notwithstanding the person's stated intention to comply, is simply that, 'it's just a bit too soon'. A related, common justification is, 'you're still not one hundred per cent/back to your baseline' (i.e., the person still has some symptoms). Such comments seem to be at odds with the MHA's intended focus on personal rather than clinical recovery and the recognition in the MHT's own guidance materials (2014, p. 22) that 'the end point of compulsory treatment within a recovery-oriented model focused on personal recovery may be considerably earlier than clinical recovery or a complete clinical resolution of symptoms.'

It is hard to see how many of these commonly used explanations justify a finding that a person who is expressing an intention to voluntarily comply with treatment cannot be treated in that less restrictive way, particularly when the mental health principles are considered. It may be that MHT members fall back on such stock explanations and justifications because they feel they are less disheartening for the person to hear than that their evidence and stated intention to comply are not accepted or believed. However, defaulting to such comments compromises transparency and natural justice, is frustrating for those who want to understand how the MHT reached its decision, and can negatively impact on the person's dignity and sense of self.

Applications for electroconvulsive treatment

As noted above, if a person who is subject to a treatment order makes an informed decision to refuse a particular treatment, their decision may be overridden by the authorised psychiatrist. However, in the case of electroconvulsive treatment (ECT) or neurosurgery for mental illness, the MHA requires the person's informed refusal to be respected.

Prior to July 2014, authorised psychiatrists could decide whether ECT should be administered to an involuntary patient (MHA 1986, s 73(3), (4)); however, since then, the MHT has had jurisdiction over compulsory ECT. Unless the person provides informed consent, ECT can only be administered to an adult on a treatment order if the MHT grants the authorised psychiatrist's application for ECT (MHA s 92(1)). To do this, the MHT must be satisfied that:

- the person does not have the capacity to give informed consent; and
- there is no less restrictive way for them to be treated (MHA s 96(1)).

As noted above, the MHA provides a definition of 'capacity to give informed consent', a presumption of capacity and principles to guide its assessment.

In 2015–2016, the MHT granted 88% of all 706 ECT applications that came before it (MHT, 2016, p. 22). Of the 12% that were refused, 56% were refused because the MHT found that treatment could be provided in a less restrictive manner, 40% because the person 'ha[d] the capacity to give informed consent,' and the remaining 4% because the MHT 'was provided with insufficient information to make a decision' (MHT, 2016, p. 22). Those latter two categories together constitute just 5% of all ECT applications, which means that the MHT was satisfied the person lacked capacity to make an informed decision about ECT in 95% of all applications that came before it.

MHDL lawyers are only able to appear in around 9% of ECT applications.[13] When surveyed, the lawyers reported either 'quite often' or 'very frequently' arguing in these hearings that the MHT could not be satisfied that the person lacked capacity to make an informed decision about ECT (whether or not the second criterion was also disputed), and that these arguments were often accepted. In 2015–2016, the MHT only granted 54% of ECT applications in which an MHDL lawyer appeared (it refused a third and adjourned a further 13%). Rather than simply deferring to the treating service's evidence about incapacity, we find that – at least when a lawyer is present – the MHT engages more directly in an assessment of incapacity in ECT hearings than VCAT does in GAA hearings.

Where the incapacity criterion is found not to be met, MHDL lawyers reported it was most often because the person positively demonstrated their ability to make an informed decision during the hearing (which is not strictly required). However, in many cases, such as Con's below, the MHT accepted that the service had taken insufficient steps (such as not providing or explaining relevant information) to put the person in a position in which their (in)ability to consent could be properly assessed. Failure to do this is inconsistent with both the statutory requirements and the Chief Psychiatrist's clinical guideline on ECT (Department of Health and Human Services, 2016).

Box 4.5 Con's case

A hospital made an ECT application for Con. Con had received ECT some years ago, which had to be ceased because of serious side effects. Because of this experience, he opposed the hospital's proposal to try ECT again. The hospital asserted that Con, who had a chronic illness, lacked capacity to make the decision. During the hearing, the lawyer established that the hospital had made only very limited efforts to engage Con in a discussion about the proposed ECT. Significantly, they had not informed him or his family that the proposed ECT would be administered unilaterally, rather than bilaterally as he had previously experienced, and so would be less likely to cause side effects. Upon learning this new information during the hearing, Con stated that he was now willing to give further consideration to ECT, because he was motivated to leave hospital as soon as possible. The MHT concluded that it could not be satisfied at that time that Con lacked capacity and dismissed the application, allowing Con to make his own decision about ECT.

These decisions demonstrate a strong respect for the specific processes which parliament prescribed to give effect to the principle that 'persons receiving mental health services should be involved in all decisions about their... treatment and recovery and be supported to make, or participate in, those decisions, and their views and preferences should be respected' (MHA s 11(1)(c)). Even though – once those processes are complied with – a further ECT application may be brought and potentially granted, it is nevertheless important that the proper process is respected.

It is perhaps unsurprising that people who are able to mobilise legal representation for their ECT hearing quickly are found to have capacity at higher rates than those who are unrepresented. However, the presence of legal representation should not significantly affect rates of MHT refusals based on insufficient information or non-compliance with proper processes because they are independent factors. Comparing the frequency with which this argument is accepted when MHDL lawyers appear with the MHT's very high rate of positive findings of incapacity across all hearings raises questions about how thoroughly the MHT examines this criterion in the 91% of ECT hearings at which MHDL lawyers do not appear.

Conclusion

While it is acknowledged that there is considerable variability between the approaches of individual VCAT and MHT members (most MHDL lawyers surveyed 'strongly agreed' that members vary significantly in their approach to the application of the law) and that both tribunals generate a range of well-reasoned, rights-respecting decisions, this chapter focused on the common practices which MHDL lawyers observe and seeks to cast light on those decisions in which it is not entirely clear how the law was applied to justify the restrictions imposed on the person's autonomy. The examination revealed:

- limited explicit consideration or exploration of decision-making capacity, except in ECT hearings at which a lawyer is present;
- a tendency to defer to clinical opinion; and
- an orientation towards outcomes, with undue weight being placed on a person's perceived best interests or concern for their future wellbeing and avoidance of risk beyond the strict parameters of the regimes.

Our experiences support the research of others (e.g., Carney et al., 2011; Diesfeld, 2003; Freckleton, 2010; Peay, 1989; Perkins, 2003) who note the tendency of MHTs to have regard to, or even rely on, de facto criteria rather than the express legislative criteria in reaching decisions. This space between the law as written and as practised on the ground raises questions about the role of tribunals in attempting to ensure people lead 'good' lives. It also raises questions about the consequent justifiability of the interventions, as the intended balance between individual rights and beneficence and/or protection which parliament set down is disrupted when tribunals fail to strictly uphold it.

While more comprehensive reform to increase the human rights compatibility of the regimes would be desirable, the likelihood of consistent, rights-respecting practices within the existing GAA would at least be improved by having a statutory definition of incapacity supported by clear principles and a process for assessing it. As we have found with the MHT's new ECT jurisdiction, these help guide decision-makers in their task and provide an objective reference to which they can be held to account. However, while this is important, such statutory guidance is not, in itself, sufficient.

Although considerably higher than the attendance rate in GAA matters, only 58% of patients attended their MHT hearings in 2015–2016 (MHT, 2016, p. 30). Low rates of attendance seriously compromise the ability of tribunals to properly assess a person's capacity, understand their wishes and give effect to the well-intentioned statutory principles which are intended to underpin each decision in practice. Even if they do attend, it is challenging for many people subject to applications or orders under these laws to effectively represent themselves and demand compliance with the law. Accordingly, the even lower rates of legal representation in these jurisdictions[14] is a further concern. Measures that could help address these issues include:

- requiring people to opt out of, rather than into, GAA reassessment hearings;
- requiring both tribunals to satisfy themselves that the person is aware of the hearing and their right to attend, and has made an informed decision not to attend, before proceeding in their absence;[15]
- adopting listing practices that allow people time to prepare and engage legal representation; and
- increasing funding to expand specialist legal services.

Until such systematic changes are made to meaningfully engage and enhance the direct participation of people at the heart of these hearings, the treatment of (in)capacity in these regimes is likely to remain inconsistent and problematic in practice.

Notes

1 I gratefully acknowledge the input of my colleagues who shared their experiences and provided feedback in the development of this chapter. VLA has authorised the use of its data, but the views expressed herein do not necessarily represent VLA's views.
2 VLA is an independent statutory authority that provides free and affordable legal help to Victorians, particularly those who are socially and/or economically disadvantaged.
3 The survey comprised 72 questions, which predominantly asked the lawyers to anonymously rate, based on their practice experience, the extent to which they agreed or disagreed with various propositions or how frequently (they perceived that) a particular situation occurs. It was completed in July 2016 by 12 of the 16 lawyers then working in MHDL. All MHDL lawyers were also provided with an opportunity to comment on the draft paper prior to finalisation.

4 According to VLA's data, in 2015–2016 we appeared in around 16% of all MHT hearings and 1% of VCAT hearings examining whether the criteria for a guardianship or administration order applied. Whether we appear is determined by whether the person has requested our assistance, our service eligibility guidelines for the particular matter (which may include consideration of the prospective merits of the matter, and any priority factors which would mean the person would struggle to represent themselves effectively) and our capacity to assist.

5 The MHT produced statements of reasons following only 3.5% (243) of the 6886 hearings at which determinations were made during 2015–2016 (MHT, 2016, p. 15), of which 165 are publicly available on Austlii (www.austlii.edu.au). Despite VCAT conducting almost 13,000 hearings relating to guardianship and administration orders in 2015–2016 (VCAT, 2016, p. 36), only 15 of these decisions are publicly available on Austlii.

6 MHT statements of reasons typically include a statement that they are not intended to be a detailed record of all material provided or issues discussed during the hearing.

7 All names used in the case studies are pseudonyms and any identifying details have been removed or altered.

8 State Trustees is a state-owned, public company which is appointed as the administrator under most administration orders.

9 The Public Advocate is an independent statutory role established to promote the rights and interests of people with disability in Victoria.

10 As noted at 4 above, MHDL appeared in around 1% of all 2015–2016 VCAT hearings examining whether the criteria for a guardianship or administration order applied. Some further representation would have been provided by other lawyers, but VCAT does not report on the rates of legal representation in GAA matters.

11 The Disability Act introduced a new legal mechanism, a supervised treatment order (STO), to authorise the detention and compulsory treatment of persons with intellectual disability who pose a 'significant risk of serious harm' to others. The concept of incapacity is directly incorporated into the fourth criterion for an STO: 'the person is unable or unwilling to consent to voluntarily complying with a treatment plan to substantially reduce the significant risk of serious harm to another person' (Disability Act s 191(6)(d)). This means that, unless the person is refusing to comply with the treatment plan, it must be established that their acquiescence or willingness to comply falls short of the legal standard for informed consent, rendering the person 'unable… to consent'. In an early and influential case, VCAT rejected the accepted interpretation of a near-identical phrase in MHA 1986 to require a higher – and thus harder to satisfy – standard when it applies to people proposed for compulsory treatment under the Disability Act. In doing so, VCAT sought to ensure that people with intellectual disability are not 'deprived of the benefits' (*MM (Guardianship)* [2008] VCAT 1282, [41]) of the compulsory treatment program or, importantly, of the scrutiny and oversight which the Disability Act was designed to provide.

12 In an unreported decision in 2013, the president of the then Mental Health Review Board (now president of the MHT) held that 'risk to self or others… was only one of five issues the Board needed to consider, and if [the person] could [consent] and was consenting to necessary treatment for [their] mental illness [they] must be discharged [from the treatment order] *even if the identified risks were high*' (emphasis added).

13 The low representation rate for ECT hearings is primarily due to the MHT's fast listing of ECT applications: in 2015–16, 50% of ECT applications were heard within one day of the application being made and 72% within two days (MHT, 2016, p. 24). This limits the opportunity for people to seek representation and for

lawyers to respond. It is not due to MHDL applying stringent guidelines or screening for merit; provided the person can give us instructions and we have the capacity to assist, we will appear for any person facing an ECT application.

14 MHDL lawyers appeared in around 16% of all MHT hearings in 2015–2016 (using VLA data), and other lawyers collectively appeared in a further 1–2% (MHT, 2016, p. 31). For legal representation in GAA matters, see 10 above.

15 The MHT's predecessor, the Mental Health Review Board, was required to satisfy itself that the person decided not to appear 'of [their] own free will' (MHA 1986, s 26(2)) but this requirement was not replicated in MHA 2014.

References

Callaghan, S., & Ryan, C. (2016). An evolving revolution: evaluating Australia's compliance with the Convention on the Rights of Persons with Disabilities in mental health law. *University of New South Wales Law Journal* 39(2), 596–624.

Carney, T., Tait, D., Perry, J., Vernon, A., & Beaupert, F. (2011). *Australian Mental Health Tribunals: Space For Fairness, Freedom, Protection & Treatment?*Adelaide: Law and Justice Foundation of NSW.

Department of Health and Human Services (2016). *Electroconvulsive Treatment: Chief Psychiatrist's Guideline*. Melbourne: Victorian Government.

Diesfeld, K. (2003). Insights on 'insight': the impact of extra-legislative factors on decisions to discharge detained patients. In K. Diesfeld & I. Freckleton (Eds.), *Involuntary Detention and Therapeutic Jurisprudence: International Perspectives on Civil Commitment* (pp. 359–382). Aldershot: Ashgate.

Freckleton, I. (2010). Extra-legislative factors in involuntary status decision-making. In B. McSherry & P. Weller (Eds.), *Rethinking Rights-based Mental Health Laws* (pp. 203–230). Oxford: Hart.

Mental Health Tribunal (2014). *A Guide to Solution-focused Hearings in the Mental Health Tribunal*. Melbourne: Mental Health Tribunal.

Mental Health Tribunal (2016). *Mental Health Tribunal 2015/2016 Annual Report*. Melbourne: Mental Health Tribunal.

Office of the Public Advocate and State Trustees (2017). *Administration Guide: A Guide for People Appointed as Administrators under the Guardianship and Administration Act 1986*. Melbourne: Office of the Public Advocate.

Peay, J. (1989). *Tribunals on Trial: A Study of Decision Making under the Mental Health Act 1983*. Oxford: Clarendon Press.

Perkins, E. (2003). *Decision-making in Mental Health Review Tribunals*. Gateshead: Athenaeum Press.

Victorian Civil and Administrative Tribunal (2015). *VCAT 2014–15 Annual Report*. Melbourne: Victorian Civil and Administrative Tribunal.

Victorian Civil and Administrative Tribunal (2016). *VCAT 2015–16 Annual Report*. Melbourne: Victorian Civil and Administrative Tribunal.

Victorian Law Reform Commission (VLRC) (2012). *Guardianship: Final Report 24*. Melbourne: Victorian Law Reform Commission.

Legislation

Disability Act 2006 (Vic)
Guardianship and Administration Act 1986 (Vic)

Mental Health Act 1986 (Vic)
Mental Health Act 2014 (Vic)
Severe Substance Dependence Treatment Act 2010 (Vic)
Victorian Civil and Administrative Tribunal Act 1998 (Vic)

Cases

McDonald v Guardianship and Administration Board [1993] 1 VR 521
MM (Guardianship) [2008] VCAT 1282
Patrick's Case (2011) 39 VR 373
XYZ v State Trustees Ltd (2006) 25 VAR 402

Chapter 5

Capacity does not reside in me

Cath Roper

Psychiatrists deem me to 'lack capacity' to consent to treatment, which means my rights to refuse treatment are removed. Instead of protecting me from violence, the state has removed my ability to protect myself from its violence: the violence of separation from loved ones, of not being believed, curtailed freedoms, the physical violence of administration of unwanted injections and pills, the violent 'take- downs' and seclusions ... Then, psychiatry rebadges this violence as actions necessary for my health and well being.

This chapter investigates the ethical situation of people treated under the *Mental Health Act Victoria 2014* (MHA), with a particular focus on how paternalism interacts with capacity to consent to treatment (mental capacity). The two main ethical principles the MHA infringes are *autonomy*, because the person cannot refuse treatment, and *bodily integrity*, through the administering of treatment to the body without consent. I conclude the MHA places people in ethical peril from which other real world negative consequences flow such as potential de-humanisation and what I term 'existential violence'.

It is argued that consumers' autonomy is undermined in the MHA in two main ways. First, if a person is compulsorily treated, the authorised psychiatrist has ultimate say over treatment decision-making, and not the person and their loved ones. Second, decision-making under the MHA is from an objective 'best interests' outcome standard, and not based on subjective standards incorporating a person's underlying values and goals, wishes and preferences, despite lip service in the principles of the MHA. I argue that the MHA has not incorporated the intent of the United Nations Convention on the Rights of Persons with Disabilities (CRPD) and its focus on the provision of support in decision-making.

If the State overrides my autonomy and bodily integrity, these are ethical wrongs, potentially with serious, multiple and ongoing consequences, and they are a matter for regret, regardless of justification, or otherwise, for compulsory treatment. To do better and ameliorate negative consequences, we must first acknowledge and regret these wrongs. Following the spirit of the CRPD is proposed as a positive and ethical way forward.

Background

The Mental Health Act Victoria, 2014

In 2008, the Mental Health and Drugs Division of the Department of Health, Victoria commenced a review of the then *Mental Health Act 1986*, aiming for compliance with obligations under Victoria's Charter of Human Rights and Responsibilities (Parliament of Victoria, 2006) and with the CRPD (United Nations, 2006), to which Australia became a signatory in 2008 (Rees, 2009). A draft exposure bill was developed subsequent to consultation processes and debated in the Victorian Parliament. In 2014, the *Mental Health Act 2014* (Vic) came into effect. The new *Mental Health Act* was heralded as progressive, particularly concerning people's rights to refuse treatment, receive support to make decisions and to have those decisions respected. Underpinning principles included recovery concepts, that people should be allowed to make decisions involving 'a degree of risk' (MHA s 11, 1(d)), and to have their 'rights dignity and autonomy respected and promoted' (MHA s 11, 1 (e)). A guiding tenet of the new MHA was to provide services to consumers in the least restrictive manner.

Components and provisions of the Mental Health Act

Measures were introduced to embed supported decision-making in the new MHA. These include presumption of a person's 'capacity to consent to treatment', a person being able to nominate someone who can represent their interests if they are temporarily unable to do so, writing an advance statement setting out treatment preferences, obtaining a second opinion and accessing independent advocacy. However, the MHA still allows for substitute decision-making in which the psychiatrist has authority to override people's treatment preferences. Advance statements under the MHA have no legal weight, nominated persons' contributions can be ignored and the MHA outweighs other health-related law. For example, the MHA would override a power of attorney for medical treatment I might have made (which would normally allow loved ones to make decisions based on my wishes) and it would override the *Medical Treatment Act* (Vic) so a Refusal of Treatment Certificate obtained under that Act has no bearing. Substitute decisions are made using a medically driven outcome standard (based on what is considered medically best, not on what the patient might have decided). It is even possible for a person's treatment decisions to be overridden despite them being deemed to have the 'capacity to consent to treatment' (Callaghan & Ryan, 2016). Thus, there are no autonomy-based principles guiding decision-making available under the MHA.

How does the Mental Health Act work?

The Act introduced a Mental Health Tribunal to oversee compliance with the Act and to hear and determine such issues as the making of treatment orders, and applications to perform electroconvulsive treatment where it is determined the patient does not have capacity to consent. I can be made subject to an assessment order (AO) if I appear to have a 'mental illness' which appears to need immediate treatment. The AO can occur in the community or an inpatient setting. I must be assessed by an authorised psychiatrist as soon as possible, but during this period I can refuse treatment unless it is considered urgent to prevent harms to myself or others. While an authorised psychiatrist can make an application for a compulsory treatment order, the Tribunal makes the decision.

United Nations Convention on the Rights of Persons with Disabilities

The CRPD has been hailed as a paradigm shift, away from a 'medical model' of disability of locating 'deficits' within an individual, towards a 'social model' in which disability is understood as the interaction between a person's impairment and social barriers, be they attitudinal, or environmental (Beresford, 2002). The social model turns our attention to the role society has in being able to guarantee the human rights and citizenship of people with disabilities on an equal basis with others through, for example, laws and policies (Morrissey, 2012). The purpose of the CRPD is to 'promote, protect and ensure the full and equal enjoyment of human rights and fundamental freedoms of all persons with disabilities and to promote respect for their inherent dignity' (United Nations, 2006, art. 1). The CRPD includes people with 'psycho-social' disabilities in its definitions of disability.

Of particular interest here is Article 12 of the CRPD, which describes 'legal capacity' as having both legal standing and legal agency: being a person before the law and being able to act within and enjoy the protections of legal frameworks (McSherry & Wilson, 2015). The CRPD, specifically Article 12, introduced the idea that with support, people with disabilities could retain 'legal capacity'. 'The premise of supported decision-making, as articulated by the disability community, is that everyone has the right to make their own decisions and to receive whatever support they require to do so' (Carter, 2009, p. 9). Supported decision-making therefore recognises that friends, families and others in a person's network may be part of decision-making. This was a move away from traditional conceptions of capacity as a cognitive ability, or attribute residing in the person, that could be tested on a pass/fail basis ('mental capacity'). Traditional conceptualisations of capacity contain a bias against people with psychiatric disabilities, often leading to infringements on their 'legal capacity' because it is assumed they do not know what is a right decision or what is in their best interests (Pathare & Shields, 2012).

Miranda Fricker's (2007) concept of 'testimonial injustice' is useful: 'Testimonial injustice occurs when prejudice causes a hearer to give a deflated level of credibility to a speaker's word' (p. 1). In our case: what mad people say is doubted and their 'mental capacity' is often judged as a marker as to whether they should be able to make their own decisions.

This becomes apparent when I disagree with the proposed treatment; then I am thought to lack 'insight' and 'capacity'. Thus the type of decision I make may be taken as a marker for my 'mental illness'. If only I were in possession of my faculties, I would see that the proposed treatment was necessary.

Similar to the social model of disability, however, capacity could be regarded as occurring between people and related to the accessibility of resources and availability of opportunities.

> That people have different decision-making abilities should not in and of itself be determinative of recognition of their legal capacity. Different decision-making abilities can be turned into decision-making *capabilities* with appropriate decision-making supports and accommodations sufficient to exercise legal capacity.
>
> (Bach & Kerzner, 2010, p. 19).

These examples expand traditional ideas about consent, decisional capacity and decision-making, highlighting that decision-making is capable of being *produced*: it is relational and contextual. The MHA, however, represents a missed opportunity to deeply engage with the implications of the CRPD. Specifically, conventional medical model notions of 'mental capacity' are not sufficiently challenged in the MHA. The Act does not invigorate mental health practice as it might have because it fails to fully embrace the new, broader definitions of 'legal capacity', which would incorporate human rights and citizenship, inspired by the CRPD, and would focus practice on the facilitation of supports and networks so individuals could retain legal capacity.

Although some language which would be consistent with the intention of the CRPD is retained, particularly in the Principles section of the MHA (such as autonomy, preferences, 'degree of risk'), it is conceptually thin, offering little guidance for practices that would challenge the 'best interests' approaches that lead to risk-averse, overly paternalistic substitute decision-making. Even taking the MHA's narrowed conception of 'capacity' ('capacity to consent to treatment'), Brophy, Ryan, and Weller (Chapter 2, this volume) and Fritze (Chapter 4, this volume) note in this volume that Tribunal hearings about treatment orders do not routinely make reference to capacity and even when they do, there is little evidence in documentation of the weighing up that should occur between capacity determinations on the one hand and the principle of providing care in the least restrictive setting on the other.

The MHA allows the undermining of consumer decision-making and onslaughts on autonomy and is not in consort with the spirit of the CRPD, especially concerning the application of ideas related to legal capacity that could have been drawn on to challenge prevailing culture of risk-averse, best interests-driven mental health services.

The intrinsic value of bodily integrity and autonomy

Bodily integrity

Bodily integrity, like autonomy, has intrinsic value and is fundamental to human dignity. 'The right to bodily integrity is a fundamental right that speaks to the notion of privacy, human dignity, and respect. It does not evaporate when individuals lose the capacity to make decisions as autonomous agents' (Maschke, 2003, p. 257). Bodily integrity is violated in any circumstance in which treatment is given against the expressed wishes (competent or otherwise) of a person. That the health or safety of a person may be protected in so doing does not change the violation.

Autonomy

Traditionally, autonomy is given high value in Western thought about morality and about health care decision-making. John Harris (1985) explains that demonstrating the principle of respect for persons means having respect for what others want to do with their lives, and the self-determined choices and decisions they wish to make in regard to their own lives because:

> autonomy is ... part of what it is to value life. For whatever it is that makes life worth living for us, and however much this differs from what makes life valuable for others, our life would cease to be of value to us to the extent that we were prevented from pursuing those things, whatever they are, that we want to pursue.
>
> (p. 200)

Within this conception of the value of autonomy is the idea that being able to live our life as we see fit is deeply connected to the meaning and worth our life has for us. It is a person's freedom to pursue their own ideas of 'the good' that gives meaning and worth to their own life. Human capacities for choice, deliberation and reflection make it possible for individuals to develop their own conception of 'the good' and to become the people they wish to be (Buchanan & Brock, 1989). In this conception, autonomy is inherently valuable because it is deeply connected to what makes life itself and the living of it valuable.

Autonomy is accorded value not solely because of what it is able to bring about (instrumental value), but has value in and of itself (Buchanan & Brock, 1989; Coggon, 2007; Goldman, 1999; Young, 1986). Intrinsic to autonomy are ideas about moral personhood, and being the self-determining agents of our own lives, making our own decisions and choices, is linked to our sense of satisfaction, dignity and self-esteem (Young 1986). Similarly, autonomous choice enables us to be held accountable for our actions, and take pride in what we do (Coggon, 2007). In contrast, the MHA sets up oppressive conditions under which violence occurs and people's autonomy, bodily integrity and even sense of self are violated.

Next I turn to the concept of paternalism deployed to provide justification for the circumstances under which this violence and violation is made lawful.

Paternalism

Gerald Dworkin (1971) defines paternalism as 'interference with a person's liberty of action justified by reasons referring exclusively to the welfare ... of the person being coerced' (p. 182). The moral concern with paternalism, as noted by Buchanan (2008) is that 'the presumption that one is right, and therefore justified in seeking to override other people's judgment, constitutes treating them as less than moral equals' (p. 15).

Paternalism and 'protection' are powerful motivations for the state in providing the overall ethical justifications for the existence of separate mental health laws. In part, the justification may not seem problematic because the MHA operates within a social context in which biomedical explanations for mental health problems hold sway, to the exclusion of other explanations. From this perspective there looks to be an unassailable logic in acting in the best interests of vulnerable people by legally ensuring that 'beneficial' psychiatric treatment can be given to them, although the same argument is not made in the case of physical health. Since it is not generally known that people governed by the MHA cannot refuse treatment, the violence of compulsory treatment is likely to remain invisible. Even if the violence were to be seen, under a medical paradigm, any ethical peril and human rights issues would likely be disappeared into justifications of beneficence. A product of the dominant Western medical approach to madness and distress is other explanatory models and successful alternative approaches for being with people such as voice hearing groups and mutual peer support are similarly, largely invisible 'out there'.

Buchanan (2008) enunciates three ways that paternalism is affected:

> Paternalism is the usurpation of decision-making power, by preventing people from doing what they have decided, interfering in how they arrive at their decisions, or attempting to substitute one's judgment for theirs, expressly for the purpose of promoting their welfare.
>
> (p. 15)

This definition of how paternalism might operate is of interest to this discussion. Under the MHA, all three forms of interference are common: I can be prevented from doing what I have decided (e.g., refraining from taking neuroleptic medication); I can be manipulated into narrowed choices (e.g., through not being given all the information pertinent to my decision, or by being given targeted information pointing me to a particular choice); and ultimately the psychiatrist can make treatment choices on my behalf as the substitute decision-maker (regardless of my capacity to consent). It should be noted that psychiatric treatments are not benign – they lower life expectancy, increase our risk of metabolic syndrome, leading to greater susceptibility to diabetes, cancers, stroke, heart disease (Lawrence, Hancock, & Kisely, 2013). The next section considers the conditions by which autonomy can be hampered or might flourish.

Conditions for autonomy

Nuanced understandings of autonomy can be rendered with a conception that includes the context in which it is exercised (or interfered with). Recent developments in feminist thought have challenged traditional Western notions of autonomy as 'individualistic' and 'atomised', instead repositioning autonomy as socially situated and relational (Friedman, 2003). Such thinking helps us to understand more about how conditions of oppression affect autonomy. Similar to ideas taken up in the social model of disability, such conceptions of autonomy emphasise ways in which environments can enable or disable.

Friedman (2003) observes that 'a disabling social context can obstruct someone's capacity to pursue her goals, ambitions and dreams' (p. 18). She argues that autonomy requires 'the absence of *effective* coercion, deception, manipulation, or anything else that interferes significantly with someone's behaving in a way that reflects her wants and values ...' (Friedman, 2003, p. 5). For Friedman, autonomous action also depends on having a significant array of opportunities reflecting what matters deeply to the person. Conditions should not limit her choices to the point where her values cannot be expressed or acted on.

For Oshana (1998), social and psychological security are inherent conditions for autonomy and include that individuals can defend themselves against (or be granted defence against) psychological or physical assault when necessary, and that individuals can pursue interests and needs different from those who may have influence or authority over them.

Taking into account the conditions under which autonomy operates helps to reflect on how, once we have been psychiatrised, many of us internalise oppressive cultural ideologies, exposing us to an internal tyranny of 'sanity' in which the only allowable way to make meaning of our distress/madness is medical, and the range of allowable behaviours shrink as we learn the exhausting arts of self-monitoring and censorship. Our sense of self crumbles, our way of being in the world, what we know, how we make meaning, is disparaged and wrong. The extent to which we are able to be truly autonomous becomes questionable.

The next section examines in more detail forms of ethical peril experienced by people subject to the MHA, and sets out how the state causes individuals subject to the MHA to be deprived of social and psychological security. Rather than protecting us as citizens, the state violates our bodies and deprives us of the necessary conditions for autonomy, subjecting us to what I term: 'existential violence'.

Ethical peril under the Mental Health Act

Potential de-humanisation

There is a particular vulnerability when the authority one has over one's own body and the ability to have one's decisions respected is denied. Under such circumstances, it is imaginable that this attitude could translate into a failure to show respect for persons. Nussbaum (1999) describes the denials of autonomy and of subjectivity as two of seven components of dehumanisation and objectification. Denial of subjectivity involves treating the person as though their experiences and feelings can be neglected. Taking a further step, there is a danger of dehumanisation, defined as the 'process of denying essential elements of "humanness" in other people and perceiving them as objects or animals' (Lammers & Stapel, 2010, p. 113). Dehumanisation is associated with misuse of power. There is a *particular* effect that comes about through thinking of a person as irrational, incompetent or mindless: 'if other people are understood as akin to objects or artefacts ... then they are free to be used instrumentally' (Haslam, 2006, p. 261).

Existential violence

This section returns to our 'traditional' definition of autonomy, this time describing the ethical losses incurred under the MHA which I argue amount to 'existential violence'.

First, the MHA jeopardises the principle of demonstrating 'respect for persons' (the starting point of morality). Flowing from this is a failure to recognise that I matter, and that how I live my life and the quality of my life matters. What I want to do with my life, and the self-determined choices and decisions I wish to make in regard to my own life, are not respected. In this picture, because I am prevented from pursuing those things that I want to pursue (whatever those things are and even if they are very different from what makes life worth living for another person), my life, the living of it, and the meaning I attach to it ceases to be of value or worth to me. If I do not have the freedom to pursue my own ideas of 'the good' I am also deprived of meaning and worth in my life. I cannot be the person I wish to be because my capacities for choice, deliberation and reflection are interfered with. When I am put in a position of not being the self-determining agent of my own life, I cannot make my own decisions and choices. As a consequence, I am denied a sense of satisfaction, dignity, self-esteem, the ability to take credit or pride for what I do, and to be held to account for my actions. In this picture, my free will is not acknowledged nor can I exercise it.

Interference with self-governance is made tangible in the example of a person on a community treatment order (CTO) who must regularly attend a clinic to be given an intramuscular injection. The CTO requirements create 'oppressive conditions' in a person's life on physical, psychological, perhaps even emotional levels. The person is not given a clear pathway for the restoration of decision-making control and, in many instances, interference with autonomy and bodily integrity extends over years.

Roessler (2015) finds that epistemic injustice 'damages and unsettles a person's relation to herself – to her self-worth as well as her self-knowledge, both of which are prerequisites for autonomous action' (p. 68). Conceptions of autonomy such as this enable us to appreciate how the loss of agency experienced through the long-term overriding of decision-making may even lead to a sense of being unable to trust our own motives or to an 'erasure of the self' (Killmister, 2015, p. 172).

What can be done?

The MHA engenders physical, existential and epistemic violence and violations of autonomy and bodily integrity. Philosopher and ethicist Michael Stocker writes about 'dirty hands' situations – these are acts that may be justifiable, even obligatory, but nonetheless 'wrong and shameful' (Stocker, 1990, p. 9). The act is to be done despite the 'dirty feature' and because of the dirty feature, the act is regrettable. The dirty features of dirty hands situations are serious: 'people being wronged, they and their trust, integrity and status as ends are violated, dishonoured, betrayed' (Stocker, 1990, p. 17). Stocker says that the dirty feature has to be counted – that it does not simply disappear on the grounds that it is part of a morally justifiable act. The counting and regretting of ethical losses and wrongs is a vital first step to lessening ethical endangerment, and there should be ethical spaces where such deliberations can take place.

The CRPD provides a pathway for thinking about ethical responses to people in distress that could challenge entrenched 'best interests' and risk-averse approaches. The MHA may set a low bar, but clinicians can rise above its failings by using the principles underpinning supported decision-making. Here, instead of an equation between 'my capacity to consent to treatment' and 'least restrictive setting', we might instead consider that capacity does not reside in the person, but rather, in the extent to which they have access to the resources they need to be able to decide for themselves, including the people in their networks, perhaps even avoiding the harms of the MHA in the first place. Expansive and creative ideas about varied resources and environments supportive of the diversity of people's autonomy needs should be prioritised and invested in.

Conclusion

Under the *Mental Health Act 2014*, treatment decisions can be made by an authorised psychiatrist on the basis of what is considered to be medically indicated and may not incorporate the person's underlying goals and values, or their wishes and preferences, despite these objectives appearing in the principles of the Act. The person's own conception of what is good and their own conception of wellbeing can be subordinated. This alone represents a significant attack on autonomy, which is so highly valued and protected in other areas of health. In addition, the incursions on autonomy and bodily integrity need to be noted and regretted. They lead to other real-world physical, existential and epistemic negative consequences.

The MHA has failed to take up the promise of the CRPD through adopting a narrow view of capacity and not challenging the paternalism that has historically shaped our responses to states of madness and distress. Paternalistic habits that place a psychiatrist's decision-making above a person's own wishes and preferences could be undone by adopting the concept of legal capacity into the MHA and by assuring a focus on the supports, relationships and networks that would help people to exercise their autonomy.

References

Bach, M., & Kerzner, L. (2010). *A New Paradigm for Protecting Autonomy and the Right to Legal Capacity – Working Paper*. Law Commission of Ontario. www.lco-cdo.org/en/our-current-projects/the-law-and-persons-with-disabilities/disabilities-call-for-papers-january-2010/commissioned-papers-the-law-and-persons-with-disabilities/a-new-paradigm-for-protecting-autonomy-and-the-right-to-legal-capacity/

Beresford, P. (2002). Thinking about 'mental health': towards a social model. *Journal of Mental Health* 11(6), 581–584.

Buchanan, A. E., & Brock, D. W., (1989). *Deciding for Others: The Ethics of Surrogate Decision Making*. Cambridge, NY: Cambridge University Press.

Buchanan, D. R. (2008). Autonomy, paternalism, and justice: ethical priorities in public health. *American Journal of Public Health* 98(1), 15–21.

Callaghan, C., & Ryan, S. (2016). An evolving revolution: evaluating Australia's compliance with the Convention on the Rights of Persons with Disabilities in mental health law. *UNSW Law Journal* 39(2), 596–624.

Carter, B. (2009). *Supported Decision-making Background and Discussion Paper*. Melbourne: Office of the Public Advocate, Victoria.;

Coggon, J. (2007). Varied and principled understandings of autonomy in English law: justifiable inconsistency or blinkered moralism? *Health Care Analysis* 15(3), 235–255.

Dworkin, G. (1971). Paternalism. In R. A. Wasserstrom (Ed.), *Morality and the Law.* Belmont, CA: Wadsworth Publishing Company.

Fricker, M. (2007). *Epistemic Injustice: Power and the Ethics of Knowing.* Oxford: Oxford University Press.

Friedman, M. (2003). *Autonomy, Gender, Politics.* New York, NY: Oxford University Press.

Goldman, A. (1999). The refutation of medical paternalism. In J. D. Arras & B. Steinbock (Eds.), *Ethical Issues in Modern Medicine* (5th edn). Mountain View, CA: Mayfield Publishing Co.

Harris, J. (1985). *The Value of Life.* London: Routledge and Kegan Paul.

Haslam, N. (2006). Dehumanization: an integrative review. *Personality & Social Psychology Review* 10(3), 252–264.

Killmister, S. (2015), Autonomy under oppression: tensions, trade-offs and resistance. In M. A. L. Oshana (Ed.), *Personal Autonomy and Social Oppression: Philosophical Perspectives* (pp. 161–179). New York, NY: Routledge.

Lammers, J., & Stapel, D. A. (2010). Power increases dehumanization. *Group Processes & Intergroup Relations* 14(1), 113–126.

Lawrence, D., Hancock, K., & Kisely, S. (2013). The gap in life expectancy from preventable physical illness in psychiatric patients in Western Australia: retrospective analysis of population based registers. *British Medical Journal* 346. doi:10.1136/bmj.f2539

Maschke, K. J. (2003). Proxy research consent and the decisionally impaired. *Journal of Disability Policy Studies* 13(4), 254–260.

McSherry, B., & Wilson, K. (2015). The concept of capacity in Australian mental health law reform: going in the wrong direction? *International Journal of Law and Psychiatry* 40, 60–69.

Morrissey, F. (2012). The UN Convention on the Rights of Persons with Disabilities: a new approach to decision-making in mental health law. *European Journal of Health Law* 19(5), 423–440.

Nussbaum, M. C. (1999). *Sex and Social Justice.* Oxford: Oxford University Press.

Oshana, M. (1998). Personal autonomy and society. *Journal of Social Philosophy* 29(1), 81–102

Parliament of Victoria (2006). *Charter of Human Rights and Responsibilities Act 2006 (43/2006).* Melbourne: Parliament of Victoria.

Pathare, S., & Shields, L. S. (2012). Supported decision-making for persons with mental illness: a review. *Public Health Reviews* 34(2), 1–40.

Rees, N. (2009). Learning from the past, looking to the future: is Victorian mental health law ripe for reform? *Psychiatry, Psychology and Law* 16(1), 69–89.

Roessler, B. (2015). Autonomy, self-knowledge, and oppression. In M. A. L. Oshana (Ed.), *Personal Autonomy and Social Oppression: Philosophical Perspectives* (pp. 161–179). New York, NY: Routledge.

Stocker, M. (1990). *Plural and Conflicting Values.* Oxford: Clarendon Press.

United Nations (2006). *Convention on the Rights of Persons with Disabilities.* UN Resolution *61/106.* www.un.org/development/desa/disabilities/convention-on-the-rights-of-persons-with-disabilities.html

Young, R. (1986). *Personal Autonomy, Beyond Negative and Positive Liberty.* Kent, UK: Croom Helm.

Legislation

Mental Health Act 1986 (Vic)
Mental Health Act 2014 (Vic)

Chapter 6

The impossibilities of 'bearing witness' to the violence of coercive interventions in the disability sector

Claire Spivakovsky

Tina is a 23-year-old woman who is forced to stay at home during the day, and locked in her bedroom overnight. When she gets frustrated with her situation, she is told her behaviour is unacceptable, and she is drugged to keep quiet.[1]

Jared is attending a meeting when someone spikes his water with a strong sedative. Jared notices that his water tastes off, but is reassured that everything is fine. Jared spends the rest of his afternoon being moved (against his will) to different locations around the state.[2]

Oliver is a school-aged boy who, like other children his age, sometimes needs to go into 'time out'. When Oliver is put into time out at his school, he is picked up and physically moved into a separate room away from everyone else, and then strapped into a chair that is bolted to the floor.[3]

Perhaps it is apparent from the title of this chapter that each of the above vignettes describes the real-life experience of a person with disability;[4] yet, I've purposely omitted any references to disability. I've done so in order to illustrate a point: when we remove the signifier of 'disability' from these scenarios, they read (at least to me) as something else. To me, they read as situations of domestic violence, of child abuse, and aggravated assault; of situations that would not be tolerated in general society, and situations that would (or at least, should) result in criminal charges. Except, in the case of people with disability, none of these scenarios would be considered criminal. In fact, in the case of people with disability, all of these scenarios are legally permissible. I find this disparity in law deeply troubling, and I am not the only one.

Countless disabled peoples' organisations and disability advocates have expressed concerns with the ways that 'restrictive practices' – the term used to describe the forms of coercive interventions applied in the disability service sector – have become 'a euphemism for what is often simply assault, false imprisonment and abuse' (Phillips, 2015, p. 54; see also Children with Disability Australia, 2015; Frohmader & Sands, 2015; Queensland Advocacy Incorporated, 2015). Despite these concerns, restrictive practices not only continue to be used against people with disability, but they continue to be presented as acceptable, necessary and 'therapeutic' responses to this population. The purpose of this chapter is to consider some of the reasons why these practices occupy this privileged position in relation to people with disability. To do this the chapter will explore some of the conditions that make it improbable, if not close to impossible, to not only question the apparent need for these practices in relation to people with disability, but to further bear witness to these practices as violence and abuse.

To meet its objectives, this chapter will engage with the recent, largely unanswered calls in Australia, from people with disability, their representative organisations and allies, for a Royal Commission into the violence and abuse of people with disability in institutional and residential settings. In particular, the chapter will focus on the recently completed Senate Community Affairs Reference Committee Inquiry into the Violence, Abuse and Neglect of People with Disability in Institutional and Residential Settings in Australia, considering the ways that this inquiry acted as a defining moment in the history of events leading up to the calls for a Royal Commission. Here the chapter will engage with the work of Jean-François Lyotard (1988) on 'the differend' to illuminate two key processes that contribute to the sustained reading of restrictive practices as 'non-violent' and 'non-criminal' activities. First, the chapter show how the Committee's Inquiry enabled representative organisations to make submissions that illuminated the messy catch-22 scenarios that sustain the reading of restrictive practices as necessary, non-violent interventions in the disability services sector. Second, the chapter will show how the Committee's Final Report worked to cleave the 'excess' from these accounts of violence and abuse, reinforcing new boundaries around what can be said about the use of restrictive practices as a 'necessary', 'therapeutic' intervention for people with disability, and what is allowed to be heard as violence and abuse. The chapter begins now by briefly engaging with what we already know about the kinds of conditions that disguise and/or sustain the use of coercive interventions in the disability services sector.

Compulsory able-bodiedness

Disability scholars have dedicated thousands of pages to showing us the many ways that people with disability are fundamentally devalued by society. We know, for example, that people with disability are regularly presented as both social and economic burdens (Oliver & Barnes, 2012), and as lesser (Goodley, Lawthom, & Runswick-Cole, 2014), contested (Hughes, 2009) and largely absent citizens (Prince, 2009). Indeed, Hughes (2012) proposes that the primary form of experience for people with disability has been one of 'invalidation'. And yet, while people with disability occupy this tenuous position in society – where their lives, experiences and opinions are pushed to, and at times, over the periphery – their physical presence remains an object of disproportionate fascination.

There is a 'cultural fetishism' associated with the disabled body (Goodley, 2014; Shakespeare, 1994). Indeed, as Goodley and Runswick-Cole (2011) explain, disabled bodies are fetishised in a whole host of contradictory ways: 'as vulnerable, dependent, broken, tragic, exotic, uber-different, pathological, violent' (p. 612). Why does this fetishism occur? Because this is how the figure of the 'normate' is produced (Thomson, 1997). The normate, as Thomson (1997) outlines, is 'the social figure through which people can represent themselves as *definitive human beings'* (p. 8; emphasis added); that is to say, it is the figure of 'normalcy' from which people can assume a privileged position of power in the processes and practices of normalisation. The normate is a figure that *requires* the mapping of a full array of 'deviant others' in order to both set its boundaries and neutralize its presence (Thomson, 1997). Unsurprisingly then, the normate is a figure that holds serious implications for the lives and bodies of people with disability.

As McRuer (2006) aptly explains, there is a 'system of compulsory able-bodiedness [in society, which] repeatedly demands that people with disabilities embody for others an affirmative answer to the unspoken question, "Yes, but in the end, wouldn't you rather be more like me?"' (p. 9). This demand for compulsory able-bodiedness takes different forms. We see it occurring through society's obsession with the 'personal tragedy theory' of disability (Oliver, 1986), and the incessant apparent need for people with disability to 'triumph over adversity' (Campbell, 2012). We also see it taking shape through the fear, disgust and general states of uncomfortableness that occur in the mirrored face of 'messy', 'leaky', or worse still, 'uncontrollable' bodies (Hughes, 2012; Shildrick, 2009). And, we see it in the assumptions that underlie practices like prenatal testing, and the apparent *only* decision that could ever be made by a parent who is told they will be giving birth to a disabled child (Kafer, 2013; see Chapter 9, this volume).

Placed together, all of these different iterations of compulsory able-bodiedness remind us that 'disabled people have not yet established their entitlement to exist unconditionally as disabled people' (Campbell, 2012, p. 215). Indeed, as Kafer (2013) and Kim (2017) explain, inherent to the system of compulsory able-bodiedness is the assumption that people with disability will, and indeed, *must* welcome all forms of intervention that might ameliorate their condition in some way. That is to say, people with disability are expected to accept all forms of 'treatment' that would assimilate their lives with that of the normate, and they are expected to do this regardless of any physical, psychic or ontological harms associated with receiving such putatively beneficial intervention. This is the curative, cultural imaginary of ableist society.

Of course, not all people with disability willingly, or indeed, unwillingly, ascribe to this ableist logic. It is when this 'dissent' from normalcy occurs that the law steps in.

Law's violent exceptions

As some critical disability and socio-legal scholars argue, the law plays a fundamental role in shaping the cultural imaginary (see, e.g., Spivakovsky, 2014; Chapter 7, this volume; Steele, 2017; Sullivan, 2017). The law, we propose, both carves out and enforces the boundaries of 'normality' and 'abnormality' in society. Indeed, as Campbell (2001; 2005) explains, we need to appreciate that the law *colludes* with biomedical discourse, 'fixing' and 'hardening' the ontology of disability through biomedical terms, and creating 'legal fictions' of disability that enshrine the boundaries of normalcy and entrench ableism in society. This is not, however, the only kind of relationship that law and biomedicine have forged, nor is it the only role the law plays in the lives of people with disability.

As Steele (2014) reminds us, people with disability are often subjected to forms of 'lawful violence'. That is to say, people with disability are often subjected to disability-specific forms of violence, such as the coercive intervention of 'restrictive practices', which are presented through law and legislature as 'humane', 'beneficial' and of course, utterly permissible responses to the lives, bodies and minds of people with disability. Indeed, we need to recognise that the violence of chemical, mechanical and physical restraints, forced sterilisation and seclusion that is meted out to people with disability under the guise of 'restrictive practices', are ultimately regulated by law, not prohibited by it, and thus these forms of violence and abuse take on a legal character (Steele, 2014, p. 473). As such, some scholars have begun to propose that people with disability exist in a 'state of exception' in relation to the law and its regulation of their 'lawful' violence.

In *Homo sacer: Sovereign power and bare life,* Agamben (1998) describes the 'state of exception' as: the 'zone of indistinction between outside and inside, exclusion and inclusion' (p. 181); a zone where there is an 'indistinction between violence and law: the threshold on which violence passes over the law and law passes over into violence' (p. 32); and, a zone that abandons those within it from the normal order of law, rendering them capable of being killed or subject to violence without impunity because 'everything … is truly possible' (p. 70). For Wadiwel (2017), this description:

> does not seem far from the practice of torture against people with disability [that is legally permitted] in institutional settings; on the contrary, it is disturbing to understand how close the resemblance is between Agamben's classic model of exception and the kinds of practices that some people with disability are routinely subject to in care institutions.
>
> (p. 390; for similar sentiments, see Adams & Erevelles, 2017; Weller, 2017)

And yet, unlike Agamben's classic model of exception (the European concentration camp), it is important to understand that the lawful violence against people with disability is not reserved for a specific kind of setting. Rather, as Steele (2017) proposes, lawful violence is reserved for the designation of 'disability *itself*' (p. 340, original emphasis). That is to say, in the case of people with disability, it is not that this population has been forced to enter some kind of pre-ordained 'camp' in society (e.g. an immigration detention centre, Abu Ghraib), and have subsequently become subject to the 'state of exception' that permeates its borders. Rather, in the case of people with disability, it is that the state of exception that permits lawful violence to be perpetrated against a person with disability *follows* the disabled body, distorting and reconfiguring what is made possible in sites like the school, home or day service, and turning these otherwise 'normal' or 'mundane' sites into bifurcated and multilayered sites of targeted violence (see Adams & Erevelles, 2017; Spivakovsky, 2017).

These developments in the use of law beg the question: what conditions make all of this possible? Or more precisely, what appears to be *stabilising* the lawful violence of people with disability in society across so many otherwise 'normal' sites and settings, especially when colleagues in law remind us that in general, 'the violence inside law threatens to undo law … to expose the façade of law's dispassionate reason as just that – a façade' (Sarat & Kearns, 1993, p. 6; see also Hunter, 2006)? An answer to this question can be found in analysing the recent, largely unanswered calls for a Royal Commission into the violence and abuse of people with disability in institutional and residential settings in Australia, and in particular, the role of a recently completed Senate Committee inquiry within this history of calls. It is to this history that this chapter now turns.

The unanswered calls for a royal commission

In November 2014, an Australian Four Corners report about the regular occurrences of abuse and violence in disability 'residential care houses' (i.e., group homes) gained significant public interest (Four Corners, 2014). Capitalising on this period of intrigue, a coalition of peak disability advocacy groups wrote to the Prime Minister of Australia, campaigning for a national inquiry into the violence, abuse and neglect of people with disability in all institutional and residential settings. In February 2015, this matter was referred to the Senate Community Affairs Reference Committee (the Committee) for action.

The Committee undertook a nine-month inquiry into the violence, abuse and neglect of people with disability in residential and institutional settings. The Committee's terms of reference stated that for this inquiry, 'violence, abuse and neglect' was to include (among other things) 'constraints and restrictive practices' as well as 'forced treatments and interventions' (Senate

Community Affairs Reference Committee, 2015, p. 4). The Committee received over 320 submissions from individuals and organisations about the violence, abuse and neglect of people with disability, with many submissions referring to the violence of restrictive practices.

In November 2015, the Committee released its Final Report. Here the Committee stated that 'under the guise of "therapeutic treatment", people with disability can be subjected to forcible actions that could be considered assault in any other context' (Senate Community Affairs Reference Committee, 2015, p. xxvi). The Committee then made a headline recommendation for a Royal Commission into the violence, abuse and neglect of people with disability in institutional and residential settings, noting that the Committee's own inquiry was unlikely to have fully captured the 'epidemic' of violence, abuse and neglect of people with disability experience. It was the contention of the Committee that 'only a Royal Commission with investigative power, funded and empowered to visit institutions could properly conduct an inquiry, and give full weight to the seriousness of this issue' (Senate Community Affairs Reference Committee, 2015, p. 268).

In March 2017, the Australian Government released its Response to the Committee (the Response). The Response announced that the Australian Government was not in agreement with the Committee, and did not believe that a Royal Commission was warranted. Instead, the Response stated that concerns about the violence, abuse and neglect of people with disability would be addressed through the forthcoming Quality and Safeguarding Framework associated with the current roll-out of Australia's National Disability Insurance Scheme (NDIS). While it is not entirely clear to what extent the forthcoming Quality and Safeguarding Framework will protect people with disability from violence, abuse and neglect going forward, it has been proposed that under the Framework a new NDIS complaints commissioner will be established. Amongst other things, the commissioner will be given responsibility for responding to the *inappropriate* or *unauthorised* use of restrictive practices; that is *some* of the violence, abuse and neglect the Committee identified in its Final Report, but notably, not the violence and abuse lying latent in the use of all restrictive practices (whether authorised or not). It will be the role of the NDIS complaints commissioner to refer matters relating to the inappropriate or unauthorised use of restrictive practices to the senior practitioner for further consideration and response. Should the senior practitioner have concerns about the violent, abusive or neglectful actions of specific workers or providers at this time, they are then entitled to further refer these matters to the NDIS registrar. The NDIS registrar is empowered to deregister or bar offending workers and/or providers should they see fit to do so.

Following the release of the Australian Government's Response and its propositions about the NDIS Quality and Safeguarding Framework, Disabled People's Organisations Australia (DPO Australia), a coalition of peak disability advocacy groups, reinstated the call for a Royal Commission. DPO Australia argued that the Government's alternative measure of the NDIS Quality and Safeguarding Framework was flawed, that this so-called response would only apply to a small fraction of people with disability (those 11% who are deemed NDIS eligible), and 'appears to be largely based on systems and responses that the Senate Inquiry found to be inadequate' (DPO Australia, 2017a). In May 2017, over 160 Australian academics joined this call for a Royal Commission, writing an open letter to Australia's Prime Minister, detailing why a Royal Commission is the only mechanism capable of infiltrating the closed nature of disability services (Disability Royal Commission Now, 2017). And, in June 2017, DPO Australia released a further Civil Society Statement stating that 'only a Royal Commission can provide a just response to people with disability who have been denied justice for so long', and 'people with disability in Australia deserve nothing less' (DPO Australia, 2017b).

At the time of writing this chapter, the current Australian Government, led by Prime Minister Turnbull, has not changed its position on the establishment of a Royal Commission. The Government continues to present the forthcoming NDIS Quality and Safeguarding Framework as the only mechanism needed for protecting people with disability from violence, abuse and neglect in institutional and residential settings.[5]

The 'differend' of coercive interventions as institutional violence

To me, the chronology of events presented above is indicative of the processes that maintain the violence perpetrated against people with disability in Australia under the guise of 'lawful' coercive interventions. That is to say, this chronology offers insight into the contours of the 'differend' (Lyotard, 1988) that surrounds and sustains this lawful violence.

In *The differend: Phrases in dispute*, Jean-François Lyotard (1988) explains that a differend occurs when the 'regulation' of a conflict between opposing parties 'is done in the idiom of one of the parties while the wrong suffered by the other is not signified in that idiom' (p. 9). When this occurs, Lyotard (1988) continues, the wronged party not only suffers from the original injury of the conflict, but further suffers the injustice of learning that the wrongs that they seek to voice currently 'exceed' the frames of reference for what is allowed to be said and heard. As such, Lyotard (1988) proposes that a differend represents 'the perfect crime', in that:

the 'perfect crime' does not consist in killing the victim or the witnesses ... but rather in obtaining the silence of the witnesses, the deafness of the judges, and the inconsistency (insanity) of the testimony. You neutralize the addressor, the addressee, and the sense of the testimony; then everything is as if there were no referent (no damages). If there is nobody to adduce the proof, nobody to admit it, and/or if the argument which upholds it is judged to be absurd, then the plaintiff is dismissed, the wrong he or she complains of cannot be attested.

(p. 9)

Of course, when reflecting on the chronology of events outlined above, it would be easy to argue that this 'perfect crime' took place when the Turnbull Government rejected the Committee's headline recommendation for a Royal Commission. That is to say, when the Government stated that it 'does not consider that a further inquiry is needed' because the NDIS Quality and Safeguarding Framework 'will protect the rights of people with disability and ensure where there is an incidence of abuse and neglect of people with disability it is addressed as a priority' (Australian Government, 2017, p. 5), the Government epitomised the process of regulating a conflict 'under the idiom of one party'. Indeed, when the Government made these claims about the kinds of protections offered by the NDIS Quality and Safeguarding Framework, it effectively rendered any renewed calls for a Royal Commission 'absurd', and any further accounts of the violence and abuse people with disability have experienced prior to the rollout of the NDIS as 'excessive' (i.e., exceeding the limits of what needs to be heard under this idiom). And yet, what I would like to propose in this chapter is that while the actions of the Turnbull Government are reflective of the differend that surrounds the violence of restrictive practices, and indeed, reinforce its operation in relation to people with disability, the actual perfect crime of the 'silent witness', 'deaf judge' and 'insane testimony' took shape at an earlier point in the previously described chronology of events. Indeed, I argue that this perfect crime took place during the generation of the Senate Community Affairs Reference Committee's Inquiry into the Violence, Abuse and Neglect of People with Disability in Institutional and Residential Settings. It is to the Committee's inquiry and its Final Report that this chapter now turns.

Silencing the witness: the self-perpetuating nature of restrictive practices

What is striking about the 320 submissions made to the Senate Committee's inquiry into the violence, abuse and neglect of people with disability in institutional and residential settings is the marked lack of submissions made by people with disability experiencing this violence. Indeed, of the submissions that are publicly available for review, fewer than 10 were written by a person with disability, with the remaining submissions written by organisations that represent or provide services to people with disability; parents or siblings of people with disability; and individuals who have at some stage worked in or alongside the disability sector. Accordingly, the overwhelming majority of submissions made to the Committee *speak for* people with disability, and as such, raise questions about the voice of people with disability in public forums, and the representativeness of the various 'others' who speak for them. Yet, regardless of how we ultimately decide to draw the line between the amplification and displacement of people with disability's voices in public settings, for the purposes of this chapter, the submissions by various 'others' serve two significant purposes.

First, these submissions bring the language of violence and abuse to discussions of restrictive practices, articulating the various contours of this lawful violence. The submission from Frohmader and Sands of the Australian Cross Disability Alliance (2015), for example, explains that the restrictive practices used against people with disability in the disability sector 'would be considered crimes if committed against people without disability, or outside of institutional and residential settings' (pp. 45–46). Likewise, the submission of Children with Disability Australia (2015) notes that the restrictive practices of 'locking a child in a small enclosure or denying food and drink are examples which would be defined as abuse if experienced in the family home but are frequently accepted or unquestioned in institutional settings' (p. 18). Yet, more than just voicing the violence of restrictive practices, these submissions are also important because they allow us to see the processes of silencing that surround this kind of violence. That is to say, they offer insight into the reasons why it could only ever be 'others', and not people with disability themselves, who articulate the contours of this specific kind of violence. This insight is most apparent in the submission made by Queensland Advocacy Incorporated (QAI).

The submission by QAI provides the case study of 'Tina', a 23-year-old woman who is being chemically restrained and subjected to extensive periods of seclusion by her disability residential service provider. In their submission, QAI (2015) explain that:

> Tina's behaviour arose because neither she nor her family were listened to. Tina was bored, had little meaningful activity in her life and had been isolated from the community in which she lived. The service provider showed little interest in addressing these issues when they were raised by the family. Instead, they attempted to restrict Tina's access to her family and on several occasions applied to QCAT [Queensland Civil and Administrative Tribunal] to have the public guardian appointed, as opposed to the family member. The service provider refused to acknowledge that Tina's behaviour was a form of communication (expressing dissatisfaction) and labelled Tina as difficult and prone to 'challenging behaviours' … [The service provider] made application to QCAT submitting that Tina could never live on her own, was unsafe to be in the community and needed high level use of Restrictive Practices.[6]
>
> (p. 18)

In these ways, QAI's submission offers insight into the contours of a troubling double-bind or catch-22 situation that appears to operate in the disability sector. Indeed, what the submission illuminates is how in the case of people with disability, the 'silence of the witness' does not simply occur when attempts to express dissatisfaction with treatment fall on 'deaf ears', but rather can occur when attempts to voice dissatisfaction are used to *the opposite effect* of their intended delivery. That is to say: that Tina would choose to express dissatisfaction with her treatment *only* works to prove that 'Tina could never live on her own, was unsafe to be in the community and needed high level use of Restrictive Practices'. Moreover, that Tina's family would raise concerns about her treatment *only* works to prove the apparent necessity to have a public guardian appointed for Tina to limit her contact with a family who apparently do not know how to act in her best interest. Thus, what the submission by QAI ultimately allows us to see is the self-perpetuating fallacy of restrictive practices that permeates the disability services sector, making it improbable – if not close to impossible – for people with disability to reveal the violence and abuse they experience in the form of coercive interventions.

Of course, drawing this conclusion about the impossibilities of bearing witness to violence from QAI's submission raises an important point of contention for this chapter. That is: even if we are willing to accept that the challenges people with disability make to the violence of restrictive practices sometimes works perversely to reinforce the apparent need for such mechanisms in the disability services sector, it is much harder to accept that these silencing processes would have the same, or indeed, any effect on those who are not subject to restrictive practices, but who still voice this violence. Put another way: is it not true that the catch-22 situation illuminated in Tina's case could still be undone, or at least, ameliorated by the fact that so many 'others' who are not subject to restrictive practices bore witness to this kind of violence in their submissions to the Committee (including QAI)? Perhaps. However, as stated in the introduction to this chapter, the Committee's Inquiry bears the markings of another process of silencing, one which works to cleave the 'excess' away from what can ultimately be heard about the violence of restrictive practices. It is to this second, compounding process of silencing that this chapter now turns.

Cleaving the 'excess' of violence from otherwise 'lawful' and 'therapeutic' interventions

The Senate Committee, its terms of reference and its final report are all vital to the recognition of restrictive practices as forms of disability-specific lawful violence. Indeed, not only did the Committee adopt the language of 'lawful violence' in its terms of reference, but it also dedicated a subsection of its final report to describing the contours of 'disability-specific lawful violence', and gave voice to submissions that spoke to the inherent criminality of restrictive practices. And yet – without wanting to diminish the significance of these actions by the Committee – it is my contention that the Committee has played a vital role in establishing the boundaries of the differend that encompasses and sustains restrictive practices as legally permitted violations of people with disability in Australia. To evince this argument, it is necessary to consider the different ways that the Committee pushes in its final report for the reduced use and/or elimination of restrictive practices in the three main settings where these practices are used in relation to people with disability: the disability service sector, prisons and schools.

Beginning with the disability service sector, it is pertinent to note that of the eight pages the Committee dedicates to discussing the use of restrictive practices in this sector, six are dedicated to describing the regulation that surrounds their use. They are used to describe which Australian states and territories regulate the use of restrictive practices in the disability service sector, which do not, and what kinds of gaps and inconsistencies exist between different jurisdictions' legislation.

Following this largely descriptive review of regulation, the Committee then acknowledges the development of Australia's *National Framework for Reducing and Eliminating the Use of Restrictive Practices in the Disability Service Sector*. It notes the delay in the completion of this Framework, and calls for the Framework to be completed and 'vigorously taken up across all jurisdictions as a priority' (Senate Community Affairs Reference Committee, 2015, p. 99). The Committee then promptly turns its attention to the use of restrictive practices in prisons without any engagement with the *experiences* of restrictive practices in the disability services sector. As such, it is in the two pages the Committee dedicates to discussing the use of restrictive practices in prisons that some of the subtle differences in the Committee's push to reduce and/or eliminate restrictive practices begin to become apparent.

From the beginning of its discussion about prisons, the Committee makes it clear that what is of issue with the use of restrictive practices in these settings is not the existence of restrictive practices per se, but rather the lack of regulation that surrounds their use. As the Committee explains, what makes it 'deeply concerned' is that there are people with disability in the prison system who:

> are not subject to the *same protections and safeguards* regarding restrictive practice as those in the disability service sector. This highlights the inappropriateness of detaining people with disability in facilities which are not *specifically for the purpose of delivery of therapeutic services*.
> (Senate Community Affairs Reference Committee, 2015,
> p. 101, emphasis added)

Given the framing of the problem, it is perhaps unsurprising that the Committee then recommends that the principles of the *National Framework for*

Reducing and Eliminating the Use of Restrictive Practices in the Disability Service Sector 'should apply to all institutions where people with disability are accommodated, particularly prisons' (Senate Community Affairs Reference Committee, 2015, p. 101).

Of course, there is much that could be said at this point about the way that the Committee appears to have recast the use of restrictive practices in the disability service sector when discussing their use in prisons. Indeed, to me it seems contradictory for the Committee to take issue with the inconsistent approaches different Australian jurisdictions have taken to regulating restrictive practices in the disability service sector – noting how this inconsistency can lead to breaches of fundamental human rights (Senate Community Affairs Reference Committee, 2015, p. 99) – and then propose that this same sector is somehow replete with 'protections and safeguards'. Moreover, it seems contradictory that the Committee can conclude that 'in many cases what is deemed to be a necessary therapeutic or personal safety intervention is in fact, assault and unlawful deprivation of liberty' (Senate Community Affairs Reference Committee, 2015, p. 115), while at the same time insinuating that the problem with restrictive practices occurring in prisons is that they do not occur under the banner of designated 'therapeutic' services and spaces, and therefore cannot be justified in the same way as practices in the disability service sector apparently can. However, before engaging further with what these apparent contradictions might imply about what can be said and heard about the lawfulness and violence of restrictive practices in Australia, it is necessary to bring attention to the final setting that the Committee addresses in its section on restrictive practices – schools – and the very different way restrictive practices are cast in this setting.

While the Committee dedicated eight pages to discussing the use of restrictive practices in the disability service sector, and a further two to prisons, 14 pages of its final report are dedicated to discussing the use of restrictive practices in schools. These 14 pages bear little resemblance to those that came before them. Indeed, it is only with respect to schools that the Committee:

- *gives voice* to numerous accounts of the harms and pains associated with the use of restrictive practices – providing substantial case studies of abuse, verbatim accounts from parents and children about the pain and humiliation associated with these practices, and several long and damming quotes about teachers, principals and school policies by disability advocates;
- *implicitly* questions the sanctity of restrictive practices as an acceptable form of intervention in relation to people with disability by repeatedly employing the use of scare quotes to refer to them as 'restrictive practices';

- *explicitly* asks 'why does it [restrictive practices] still happen?' (Senate Community Affairs Reference Committee, 2015, p. 114), before concluding that the ongoing use of restrictive practices in educational settings is 'without a doubt a national shame' (Senate Community Affairs Reference Committee, 2015, p. 115); and
- *invokes societal norms* for the first time, stating that restrictive practices in schools 'clearly do not meet community expectations and standards when it comes to how children – abled or with disability – are treated' (Senate Community Affairs Reference Committee, 2015, p. 114).

Given these differences in emphasis, it is perhaps unsurprising that in the case of schools, the Committee does not simply call for the completion and extension of the *National Framework for Reducing and Eliminating the Use of Restrictive Practices in the Disability Service Sector* (as it did with the disability services and the prison sectors). Rather, in the case of schools, the Committee further states that the use of restrictive practices in schools *must* be eliminated 'as a national priority', calling on the Australian Government to 'implement a zero-tolerance approach to restrictive practice in a school context' (Senate Community Affairs Reference Committee, 2015, p. 279).

To me, the different emphasis the Committee places on pushing for the reduction and/or elimination of restrictive practices in the disability service sector, prisons and schools is significant. In particular, it allows us to see the role the Committee has come to play in sub-dividing the violence of restrictive practices in Australia. That is to say, it shows us the ways that the Committee's Report cleaves the instances of disability-specific violence that are said to warrant law's immediate prohibition away from those that are only believed to require law's (tighter and more consistently applied) regulation. And, in these ways, these differences allow us to see the important role the Committee has played in determining what can ultimately be said or heard about both the violence and sustained lawfulness of restrictive practices in Australia. And yet, more than this, I would like to propose that the different emphasis the Committee places on pushing for the reduction and/or elimination of restrictive practices in the disability service sector, prisons and schools allows us to see something else. It allows us to see the system of compulsory able-bodiedness described earlier in this chapter, and the strength of the curative imaginary and ableist logics that it espouses.

It cannot be overlooked that the only time the Committee calls upon the law to prohibit restrictive practices is in relation to the one setting that is co-occupied by the figure of the normate: the school. That, for both the disability services sector and the prison – two settings reserved for the normate's array of deviant others – the Committee instead pushes to *maintain the legal character* of this form of violence. Indeed, it cannot be overlooked that in these settings designated for the normate's deviant others to occupy, what the Committee ultimately calls for is the tighter and more consistent regulation so that only the so-called 'therapeutic' parts of restrictive practices can remain unchanged, with people with disability expected to just continue accepting these forms of intervention in their lives regardless of any associated harms. Accordingly, in these ways, it is important to understand that what the Committee's report ultimately does is not just cleave the excess of law's violence from the practice of restrictive interventions. Rather, the report works to *clean* the excess accounts made by people with disability and their advocates that might otherwise be able to be used to reconnect this newly divided terrain, selectively reinstating the banner of 'therapeutic' interventions that makes stories of violence or abuse sound absurd. It is on this point that this chapter draws its final conclusion.

Conclusion

This chapter was based on the premise that restrictive practices are disability-specific forms of violence that have been enabled to appear lawful, therapeutic and necessary. The purpose of the chapter was to explore some of the conditions that stabilise these renderings of this violence. To do this, the chapter worked through the example of the recent, largely unanswered calls for a Royal Commission into the violence and abuse of people with disability in institutional and residential settings in Australia, focusing in particular on the Senate Committee's inquiry into the same topic. Here, the chapter revealed some of the contours of a differend that works to silence (either in total or in part) the testimonies of restrictive practices as unlawful and/or unacceptable forms of targeted abuse committed against people with disability. In doing so, what this chapter ultimately offers is new insight into some of the processes that work to enforce the curative imaginary of society and stabilise the ableist logics that restrict and violently prohibit people with disability from the entitlement of an unconditional existence.

Notes

1 This is an abridged case study adapted from Queensland Advocacy Incorporated (2015).
2 This example was provided to me by a disability service provider during some interviews I undertook as part of the project *Understanding and Responding to Key Issues in Disability and Mental Health Care* (see Spivakovsky (2016) for the full report).
3 This example was adapted from Children with Disability Australia (2015).
4 Throughout this chapter I use the terminology 'people with disability'/'person with disability' as opposed to 'people with disabilities'/'person with a disability'. This use of terminology is advocated by disabled peoples organisations, and recognises that disability is the result of the interaction between people living with impairments and an environment filled with physical, attitudinal, communication and social barriers, and not just one or more impairments that need to be diagnosed, categorised and hierarchised by medicine.

5 Notably, the Leader of the Opposition, Bill Shorten, has announced that the Australian Labor Party will establish the Royal Commission if elected as the next Australian Government in 2019.
6 I've purposely only provided one example here, as I am conscious of the fine line that needs to be trodden between describing the experiences of people with disability and contributing to their fetishisation.

References

Adams, D.L., & Erevelles, N. (2017). Unexpected spaces of confinement: Aversive technologies, intellectual disability, and 'bare life'. *Punishment & Society* 19(3), 348–365.

Agamben, G. (1998). *Homo sacer: Sovereign power and bare life.* Redwood City, CA: Stanford University Press.

Australian Government (2017). *Australian Government Response to the Senate Community Affairs References Committee Report: Violence, abuse and neglect against people with disability in institutional and residential settings, including the gender and age related dimensions, and the particular situation of Aboriginal and Torres Strait Islander people with disability, and culturally and linguistically diverse people with disability.* Commonwealth of Australia: Canberra.

Campbell, F. K. (2001). Inciting legal fictions: Disability's date with ontology and the ableist body of the law. *Griffith Law Review* 10(1), 42–62.

Campbell, F. K. (2005). Legislating disability: negative ontologies and the government of legal identities. In S. Tremain (Ed.), *Foucault and the government of disability.* Ann Arbor, MI: University of Michigan Press.

Campbell, F. K. (2012). Stalking ableism: using disability to expose 'abled' narcissism. In D. Goodley, B. Hughes & L. Davis (Eds.), *Disability and social theory.* London: Palgrave Macmillan.

Children with Disability Australia (2015) *Submission to the Senate Inquiry into Violence, Abuse and Neglect against People with Disability in Institutional and Residential Settings.* Melbourne: Children with Disability Australia.

DisabilityRoyalCommissionNow (2017). *Open letter from academics supports calls for a Royal Commission into violence against people with disability.* https://disabilityroyalcommissionnow.wordpress.com/2017/04/05/open-letter/

Disabled People's Organisations Australia (DPO Australia) (2017a). *Disability groups call for Royal Commission into violence against people with disability.* 27 March 2017. http://dpoa.org.au/disability-groups-call-for-royal-commission-into-violence-against-people-with-disability/

Disabled People's Organisations Australia (DPO Australia) (2017b). *Civil society statement to the Australian Government – end the violence: Call a Royal Commission into violence and abuse against people with disability.* 7 June 2017. http://dpoa.org.au/civil-society-statement-rc/

Four Corners (2014) *In Our Care.* Aired Monday 24 November 2014. Transcript available from: www.abc.net.au/4corners/stories/2014/11/24/4132812.htm

Fricker, M. (2007). *Epistemic injustice: power and the ethics of knowing.* Oxford: Oxford University Press. Retrieved 4 Jan. 2018, from www.oxfordscholarship.com/view/10.1093/acprof:oso/9780198237907.001.0001/acprof-9780198237907.

Frohmader, C., & Sands, T. (2015). *Australian Cross Disability Alliance (ACDA) submission to the Senate Inquiry into Violence, Abuse and Neglect against People with Disability in Institutional and Residential Settings.* Sydney: ACDA.

Goodley, D. (2014). *Dis/ability studies: Theorising disablism and ableism.* Routledge: London.

Goodley, D., Lawthom, R., & Runswick-Cole, K. (2014). Posthuman disability studies. *Subjectivity* 7(4), 342–361.

Goodley, D., & Runswick-Cole, K. (2011). The violence of disablism. *Sociology of Health & Illness* 33(4), 602–617.

Hughes, B. (2009). Disability activism: social model stalwarts and biological citizens. *Disability & Society* 24(6), 677–688.

Hughes, B. (2012). Civilising modernity and the ontological invalidation of disabled people. In D. Goodley, B. Hughes & L. Davis (Eds.), *Disability and social theory.* London: Palgrave Macmillan.

Hunter, R. (2006). Law's (masculine) violence: reshaping jurisprudence. *Law and Critique* 17, 27–46.

Kafer, A. (2013). *Feminist, queer, crip.* Indiana: Indiana University Press.

Kim, E. (2017). *Curative violence: Rehabilitating disability, gender, and sexuality in modern Korea.* Durham, NC: Duke University Press.

Lyotard, J. F. (1988). *The differend: Phrases in dispute.* Minneapolis: University of Minnesota Press.

McRuer, R. (2006). *Crip theory: Cultural signs of queerness and disability.* New York: New York University Press.

Oliver, M. (1986). Social policy and disability: some theoretical issues. *Disability & Society* 1(1), 5–17.

Oliver, M., & Barnes, C. (2012). *The new politics of disablement* (2nd edn). London: Palgrave Macmillan.

Phillips, J. (2015). *Committee Hansard.* Sydney, 27 August.

Prince, M. (2009). *Absent citizens: Disability politics and policy in Canada.* Toronto: University of Toronto Press.

Queensland Advocacy Incorporated (QAI) (2015) *Submission to the Senate Inquiry into Violence, Abuse and Neglect against People with Disability in Institutional and Residential Settings.* Brisbane: Queensland Advocacy Incorporated.

Sarat, A., & Kearns, T. (1993). *Law's violence.* Ann Arbor, MI: University of Michigan Press.

Senate Community Affairs References Committee (2015). *Violence, abuse and neglect against people with disability in institutional and residential settings, including the gender and age related dimensions, and the particular situation of Aboriginal and Torres Strait Islander people with disability, and culturally and linguistically diverse people with disability.* Commonwealth of Australia: Canberra.

Shakespeare, T. (1994). Cultural representation of disabled people: dustbins for disavowal? *Disability & Society* 9(3), 283–299.

Shildrick, M. (2009). *Dangerous discourses of disability, subjectivity and sexuality.* London: Palgrave Macmillan.

Spivakovsky, C. (2014). Making risk and dangerousness intelligible in intellectual disability. *Griffith Law Review* 23(3), 389–404.

Spivakovsky, C. (2016). *Key issues in disability and mental health care: Insights from a state-wide consultation into restrictive and coercive interventions.* Melbourne: Monash University.

Spivakovsky, C. (2017). Governing freedom through risk: locating the group home in the archipelago of confinement and control. *Punishment & Society* 19(3), 366–383.

Steele, L. (2014). Disability, abnormality and criminal law: sterilisation as lawful and 'good' violence. *Griffith Law Review* 23(3), 467–497.

Steele, L. (2017). Policing normalcy: sexual violence against women offenders with disability. *Continuum* 31(3), 422–435.

Sullivan, F. (2017). Not just language: an analysis of discursive constructions of disability in sentencing remarks. *Continuum* 31(3), 411–421.

Thomson, R. G. (1997). *Extraordinary bodies: Figuring physical disability in American culture and literature*. New York: Columbia University Press.

Wadiwel, D. (2017). Disability and torture: exception, epistemology and 'black sites'. *Continuum* 31(3), 388–399.

Weller, P. (2017). Mental capacity and states of exception: revisiting disability law with Giorgio Agamben. *Continuum* 31(3), 400–410.

Part III

Regulating the production of 'good', 'healthy' and 'meaningful' lives

The previous part of this book provided us with three contributions that spoke to the material impacts and lived effects of coercion. These chapters raised profound and disturbing questions about how we treat some of society's most vulnerable populations, and the harms that might be perpetrated in the name of 'beneficial', 'necessary' and 'lawful' interventions. In this third part of the book, we shift our attention outward, and consider how the rationales underpinning decisions to coercively intervene in the lives of certain populations (and not others) might also intersect with overarching and long-standing goals of governance and population management.

The chapters in this third part offer insight into the ways that social processes for producing 'good', 'healthy' and 'productive' lives are not evenly calibrated. These chapters draw attention to the ways that decisions to use coercive interventions often speak to and reinforce a range of demarcations between citizens. Indeed, the intersection between coercive interventions and the governance and division of citizenry is of direct concern in the first chapter (by Claire Spivakovsky and Kate Seear) on problem-solving courts.

Spivakovsky and Seear engage with Bacchi and Beasley's (2002) argument that social policy often produces a demarcation between 'full' and 'lesser' citizens. As Bacchi and Beasley (2002) explain, this division is typically hinged upon a dichotomy of 'control over body'/'controlled by body', justifying the illiberal treatment of those 'lesser' citizens who are believed to have 'lost control'. In their chapter, Spivakovsky and Seear show how this dichotomy of bodily control was deployed in the establishment of both Victoria's drug and mental health courts, with significant implications. Indeed, their chapter demonstrates how perceptions about the levels of choice that people with 'addiction', mental illness and/or cognitive impairment have in 'losing control', as well as beliefs about the capacity of these populations to make more 'productive' choices going forward, enables new subdivisions to form between these 'lesser' citizens. As Spivakovsky and Seear argue, these subdivisions hold serious implications for the kinds of interventions believed to be necessary for these populations in both the short and long term, and the kinds of 'meaningful' lives these populations are believed capable of maintaining. Notably, the long history of coercively governing 'good', 'healthy' and 'meaningful' ways of living is also addressed by Stephen Gray in his chapter on the Healthy Welfare Card.

The Health Welfare Card is a recently introduced form of income control in Australia, which restricts welfare recipients from purchasing alcohol and gambling products. As Gray explains in his chapter, the Healthy Welfare Card is claimed to empower welfare recipients to become healthy consumers and lead more productive lives, and is currently being trialled in three jurisdictions of Australia. These three trial sites have substantial Indigenous populations, which leads Gray to propose that the recent emergence of the Healthy Welfare Card in Australia can actually be located in the much longer colonial history of white Australia's efforts to assimilate Indigenous peoples into the mainstream through coercive measures. Indeed, what Gray's chapter allows us to see is the numerous ways that Indigenous peoples have come to be managed by government-led coercive measures over time. His chapter shows that each time governments intervene in the lives of Indigenous peoples, these coercive measures work simultaneously to undermine these populations' self-determination, while claiming to champion their empowerment and produce more productive ways of life. In these ways, Gray's chapter reminds us of how contemporary rationales for medico-legal coercive interventions can be used to reinforce other, much older processes of stratification in society. Indeed, when read together with Spivakovsky and Seear's chapter, Gray's contribution allows us to see how the assumptions about bodily control and productive choices used to justify contemporary medico-legal interventions can also be used to deflect, disguise and even neutralise the ongoing presence of racialised practices in population management. It is to this issue of neutralising other histories of intervention that the final two chapters in this part of the book speak, albeit through reference to a different population stratum.

The final two chapters in Part III turn our attention to a population which is often assumed to be lacking bodily control but rarely considered in any detail within the literature on coercive interventions: children. Linda Steele and Ian Freckelton examine the legal jurisdictions that enable courts to authorise significant medical interventions in the lives of a child. Steele focuses on the Family Court of Australia's 'welfare jurisdiction', and its use in authorising the sterilisation of young girls with intellectual disability. Freckelton explores the Western Australian Family Court's use of the *parens patriae* jurisdiction (a jurisdiction that is designed to safeguard the interests of 'those unable to protect themselves'), and considers how this jurisdiction was applied in the case of a very ill boy whose parents opposed elements of conventional medical treatment.

Both Steele and Freckelton bring light to the assumptions about health and productive choices that underpin medico-legal judgments about what constitutes the child's 'best interest'. And yet, due to their disparate targets – Steele focusing on girls with disability, and Freckelton on a boy with a serious medical condition – these chapters ultimately provide very different accounts of law. Indeed, Steele and Freckelton expose us to the very different kinds of medico-legal judgments that the legal fraternity feels comfortable in making in relation to boys and girls, and in relation to illness and disability. In doing so, Steele and Freckelton's contributions allow us to catch a glimpse of the broader processes of stratification that are often hidden within coercive interventions, showing us the ways that assumptions about bodily control, 'productive' choices and the need to employ medico-legal coercive interventions with 'lesser' citizens, can also be shaped by longstanding gendered and ableist approaches to governance and population management.

The contributions in this part of the book speak to the ways that coercive interventions reinforce a range of enduring demarcations between 'full' and 'lesser' citizens. Indeed, they allow us to understand how contemporary medico-legal concerns about bodily control can disguise, deflect and neutralise much older processes of population management. In these ways, the chapters in this part of the book enable us to locate contemporary coercive interventions within the long histories of using the powers of law and medicine to produce *particular kinds* of 'good', 'healthy', and 'meaningful' lives amongst the citizenry.

Chapter 7

Making the abject

Problem-solving courts, addiction, mental illness and impairment[1]

Claire Spivakovsky and Kate Seear

This chapter is concerned with the ways that certain 'problems' and 'solutions' of normalcy and disability become associated with, constituted by and given meaning through political, discursive representations. Specifically, we are interested in tracing how the growing number of people with cognitive impairments, mental illness and/or alcohol or other drug (AOD)[2] dependence in Australian prisons has emerged as a central 'problem' of law and justice in the past two decades, and the effects that occur when 'problem-solving' courts take shape as the logical, necessary 'solution'. To do this, we analyse the parliamentary debates surrounding the creation of two problem-solving courts in the Australian state of Victoria: the Drug Court, and the Assessment and Referral Court List (a specialist court list for people with cognitive impairments and/or mental illness). Adapting Carol Bacchi's (2009) theoretical framework for analysing policy 'problems' to the study of law, we draw out the different ways that these specialist jurisdictions have been conceptualised in political, formative debates, focusing on the 'problems' they are purportedly designed to solve, and the effects for their target populations. We reflect on the ways that these debates provide access to deep-seated presuppositions and pervasive cultural logics about agency, capacity, disability and crime, and enable certain modes of governance to take form.

The emergence of 'problem' populations and therapeutic 'solutions'

There are growing and disproportionate numbers of people entering Australian prisons who experience AOD dependence, cognitive impairments and/or mental illness. While only 15% of Australia's general population use illicit drugs (AIHW, 2011), this proportion increases to 70% for prison entrants, with many experiencing AOD dependence (AIHW, 2013). At the same time, 31% of prisoners have been treated for a mental health disorder (AIHW 2012) – approximately 2.5 times the proportion in the general population (ABS, 2010) – and somewhere between 25% (Morrell, Merbitz, & Jain, 1998) and 82% (Schofield, Butler, & Hollis, 2007) of prisoners are living with a traumatic brain injury. These figures have prompted important questions about the reasons why people experiencing AOD dependence, cognitive impairments and/or mental illness are over-represented in criminal justice systems, as well as queries about the appropriateness and effectiveness of criminal justice interventions (see Butler et al., 2005; Lamberti et al., 2001; Prins, 2011). In response to such questions, specialist, 'problem-solving' courts have emerged.

Problem-solving courts are purpose-designed, specialist jurisdictions which aim to address the underlying social, medical and/or psychological issues that are believed to underpin certain populations' contact with criminal justice systems. Derived from the therapeutic jurisprudence movement of the United States, the courts operate on the premise that law, its personnel and processes can have therapeutic effects on participants' wellbeing (Wexler & Winick, 1996). The courts aim to foster the therapeutic potential of the law by taking into consideration both the treatment and justice concerns of the accused and any victims. The result of this consideration can take several forms, including diversionary processes (that is, processes which divert people from the traditional court system, offering a chance to avoid a criminal record), and providing intensive, mandatory, medical and psychological treatments in the community.

Scholars have interrogated the development of problem-solving courts from several perspectives. Predominately, research has been evaluative in nature, measuring the courts' clinical effects (e.g., Boothroyd et al., 2005; Cosden et al., 2003), or their capacity to manage risk and reduce recidivism (e.g., Herinckz et al., 2005; McNeil & Binder, 2007; Steadman et al., 2011). Some have also investigated the consequences of merging adversarial and therapeutic court approaches, raising concerns about the extended periods of time offenders spend in contact with criminal justice systems through these approaches, and the intrusive nature of the interventions imposed (e.g. Boldt, 2002; Hannah-Moffat & Maurutto, 2012; Moore, 2007). This chapter seeks to engage with problem-solving courts in another way. Rather than focusing on the putative impacts of these courts – intended or otherwise – we are interested in tracing the different processes of 'problem' construction that have informed the development of Victoria's Drug Court and Assessment and Referral Court List, the pervasive cultural logics which inform this construction process, and the effects this has on targeted populations. To draw out these different facets, we turn to the analytical strategy of the highly influential Australian poststructuralist theorist, Carol Bacchi.

Bacchi, policy problematisation, and the law

Inspired by Michel Foucault's work on 'problematisation', Bacchi is concerned with 'thinking problematically' about policymaking. For Bacchi, policy 'problems' are not fixed or stable phenomena; they 'do not exist "out there" in society, waiting to be "solved" through timely and perspicacious policy interventions' (Bacchi & Eveline, 2010, p. 111). Rather, working with Foucault's observation that discursive and non-discursive practices produce things as 'objects for thought' (Foucault, 1988, p. 257), Bacchi proposes that policies '*give shape* to "problems"; they do not *address* them' (2009, x, emphasis original). Bacchi argues that 'problems' are constituted through and given meaning by the *representations* embedded within public policy. Bacchi thus encourages us to critically interrogate the presuppositions and conceptual logics which underpin policies and policymaking practices, unearthing the problem representations that purport to naturally 'pre-exist' the policy-making process.

Interrogating presuppositions and conceptual logics are important because, as Bacchi (2009) points out, policy representations are 'political interventions' (p. 35) which 'imagine' problems, 'in particular ways that have real and meaningful effects' (Bacchi & Eveline, 2010, p. 111). Bacchi (2009) identifies three main 'effects':

- *discursive effects* – the ways in which problem representations limit what can be thought or said;
- *subjectification effects* – the ways in which particular kinds of subjects and subject positions are discursively produced; and
- *lived effects* – the 'real' and material repercussions of these problematisations in people's lives.

To draw out problem representations and their effects, Bacchi (2009) offers an analytical strategy called 'What's the Problem Represented to be?' This strategy comprises six questions, which can be undertaken together or selectively.[3] The questions are:

1   What is the 'problem' represented to be in a specific policy or policy proposal?
2   What presuppositions or assumptions underpin this representation of the 'problem'?
3   How has this representation of the 'problem' come about?
4   What is left unproblematic in this problem representation? Where are the silences? Can the 'problem' be thought about differently?
5   What effects are produced by this representation of the 'problem'?
6   How/where has this representation of the 'problem' been produced, disseminated and defended? How has it been (or could it be) questioned, disrupted and replaced?(adapted from Bacchi, 2009, xii)

In recent years, this strategy for examining policy 'problems' has been adapted to analyses of the law (Lancaster, Seear, & Treloar, 2015; Seear & Fraser,

2014). Seear and Fraser (2014) argue that Bacchi's strategy is well suited to the study of law and legal processes, because – like policy – it is possible to:

> see the law as reflecting, and in turn re-enacting, the (always changing) values of a given society. If we read legal discourse as does Bacchi on policy, we can expose its role in formulating social problems rather than simply addressing them. Doing this allows us to create space to critically assess these formulations for their assumptions and oversights, and for the ways in which they might reinforce or exacerbate social inequalities or exclusions as much as ameliorate them.
>
> (p. 828)

In this chapter we extend this work further, analysing the pervasive cultural logics which enable specialist court systems to emerge as logical, wholly beneficial 'solutions' to the growing number of people with AOD dependence, cognitive impairments and/or mental illness entering prisons. We further consider how this process of defining 'solutions' limits what can be said about the lives of people with AOD dependence, cognitive impairments and/or mental illness, and their criminal activity. As such, our focus is not on the everyday operations of the specialist systems themselves, but on the legislative processes through which these courts came about. We explore these processes through an analysis of parliamentary debates pertaining to the development of both the Victorian Drug Court and the Assessment and Referral Court List. Such debates (including the second reading speech) enable us to access the deep-seated presuppositions and claims (both express and implied) about the purported 'true nature' of the particular 'problem' requiring this specialist response. Focusing in particular on questions 1, 2 and 5 of Bacchi's strategy, we trace a few of the effects (discursive, subjectification and lived) on the targeted populations of the courts.

The Victorian Drug Court

The Victorian Drug Court was established as a division of the Magistrates' Court by the *Sentencing (Amendment) Act 2002* (Vic). Under s4B of the *Magistrates Court Act 1989* (Vic), a proceeding can be adjourned to the Drug Court if it appears that the accused:

• might be eligible for a drug treatment order (DTO);
• resides within a postcode area covered by the Drug Court; and
• consents to the adjournment.

To be eligible for a DTO, several conditions must be satisfied (s18Z *Sentencing Act 1991* (Vic)). Among other things, the accused must be willing to plead guilty and submit to a DTO; they must not be charged with a sexual or violent offence; and crucially, the Court must be satisfied on the balance of probabilities that the accused is dependent on drugs or alcohol, and that such dependency contributed to the commission of the offence.

Agency, capacity and the criminogenic addict

The Bill to propose a Drug Court in Victoria was debated in November 2001 and February 2002. These debates reveal a consistent but internally contradictory conceptualisation of the 'addicted' subject's agency and capacity to independently make changes in their lives. Although addicts are described as having 'complex individual needs' (Hulls, *Hansard*, 29 November 2001, p. 2193), they are also constructed as largely predictable, with 'chaotic lifestyles' (Hulls, *Hansard*, 29 November 2001, p. 2191) that hinder their ability to function normally. Most often, addicts are positioned as incapable of change, rational action and/or self-control, being 'desperate and usually driven by one urge, and that is to get the next hit or whatever you would call it' (Savage, *Hansard*, 27 February 2002, p. 131). According to members of the Legislative Assembly, addicts live a life of 'despair', trapped by virtue of 'being permanently *caught in a web* of addiction' (Savage, *Hansard*, 27 February 2002, p. 131; our emphasis). These are people 'who probably will not rehabilitate for the rest of their life' (Dean, *Hansard*, 27 February 2002, p. 104).

Here, the presumed effects of addiction are represented as harmful, restrictive and devastating for the individuals so affected. Yet despite the apparently significant personal costs of addiction, the 'true problem' to be addressed by law and policy is that of addiction-fuelled crime. Indeed, the then Attorney-General Rob Hulls lamented the traditional criminal justice system's approach towards drug use and offending, suggesting that it 'punishes their offending without addressing the *cause* of that offending: drug addiction' (Hulls, *Hansard*, 29 November 2001, p. 2191; our emphasis).

Hulls' comments reveal an important set of assumptions about the 'problem' at play during the parliamentary debates of 2001–02: the notion that drug addiction is *inherently criminogenic*. Indeed, 'anti-social behaviour'[4] is described as being '*a result* of their dependency on drugs' (McCall, *Hansard*, 27 February 2002, p. 121; our emphasis); a 'reality' whereby 'this person is breaking into people's houses *because* he [sic] is a drug addict and that *will continue for so long as he* [sic] *is a drug addict*' (Dean, *Hansard*, 27 February 2002, p. 103; our emphasis). Similarly, burglary and assault are portrayed as things often done 'to get the money to provide for their drug habit' (Wells, *Hansard*, 27 February 2002, p. 125). In fact, in this account not only does criminality follow drug use and/or addiction, but a pathway of gradually increasing severity can be identified in many instances:

> Many of those who have been associated with drug dependency have moved from actions within the family circle to petty theft and more

serious crime to support their drug habits. The pattern of progression is well and truly established and can be seen in the many cases that we are all aware of.

(Stensholt, *Hansard,* 27 February 2002, p. 123)

This representation of the relationship between crime and addiction has important implications for the construction of the addict's agency. Paradoxically, addicts are largely positioned as lacking agency and the capacity for change, while being simultaneously responsible for their behaviour, and for altering it. In the following passage, for instance, offending is positioned as an 'effect' of addiction, at the same time as the addict is reprimanded for *persisting* with offending. The emphasis on *discouraging* people who use drugs from so doing, while also purportedly *deterring* addicts through the threat of future imprisonment, suggests a subject who is agentive, responsive, responsible and capable of change:

> I would hope that what we are looking for in the drug courts is the opportunity to discourage those who have not reached the stage of addiction from continuing their antisocial behaviour. We should therefore view the drug courts in the light of prevention rather than cure. They should in some ways act as part of a package of deterrents that establish that people who persist in antisocial behaviour as a result of their dependency on drugs will end up in a much more severe environment and will potentially end up serving custodial sentences behind bars for an indefinite period of time.
>
> (McCall, *Hansard,* 27 February 2002, p. 121)

In Bacchi's terms, these passages reveal how the 'problem' of addiction, drugs and drug-related crime emerged within the context of the parliamentary debates. The principal problem to be addressed is the (paradoxically, simultaneously) non-agentive/choosing subject whose poor choices have rendered them unable to bring their 'anti-social behaviour' under control.

This configuration of the addict is somewhat familiar. It is, for example, largely consistent with traditional tropes of addiction, where the subject is positioned as chaotic, false, dependent, irrational and lacking control (e.g., Fraser & Seear, 2011; Keane, 2002), while simultaneously being enjoined to action, and responsibilised (e.g., Fraser, 2004). Yet by rehearsing this familiar narrative within the context of the Drug Court's development, certain discursive and subjectification effects take hold. Not only do drug users paradoxically become simultaneously non-agentive/choosing subjects, but other ways of conceptualising their crimes are foreclosed. It is no longer possible to imagine, for example, that some 'addicts' may not partake in criminal offending, or that where they do, the origins of such offending might be either more complex or undertaken for reasons unrelated to drug use. Drugs and addiction, it would seem, are the sole/principal causes of crime and 'anti-social behaviour' because, once chosen by the subject, they become all-controlling. This is an important conceptual logic, and one which carries certain familiar repercussion in law and policy. It is to these repercussions we turn now.

Rehabilitating lesser citizens back to their full potential

Bacchi and Beasley (2002) argue that much of Australian social policy is underpinned by 'a demarcation between full and lesser citizens which hinges precisely upon assumptions about bodies' (p. 325). They propose that two kinds of political subjects are often produced through policy responses: 'those deemed to be in control of their bodies [full citizens], and those considered to be controlled by their bodies [lesser citizens]' (p. 325). Bacchi and Beasley (2002) argue that the 'control over body'/'controlled by body' dichotomy is often deployed within social policy as a means of justifying the 'illiberal treatment of some citizens' (p. 338). They propose that through locating the division of citizenship within a medicalised discourse of the body, certain constraints, restrictions and intrusions upon the 'autonomy' of citizens becomes palatable (as long as they are overseen by the medical profession). This appears to be what has taken place in the context of the development of the Drug Court.

Having rendered drugs and addiction as inherently criminogenic, and the 'addict' as controlled by this criminogenic addiction (which, at the same time, they have chosen), a neatly aligned yet highly intrusive 'solution' emerges. With its focus on finding ways to 'cure people's problems by freeing them from their addictions' (Savage, *Hansard,* 27 February 2002, p. 131) – as opposed to simply imprisoning the person for their crimes – the Drug Court is purported to simultaneously 'facilitate the rehabilitation of the offender' (Hulls, *Hansard,* 29 November 2001, p. 2192) and 'protect the community' (Hulls, *Hansard,* 29 November 2001, p. 2191) from the 'anti-social behaviours' associated with their poor choice. In other words, by drawing upon the conceptual logic surrounding bodies, control and citizenship, members of the Legislative Assembly both exclude the prospect that other forms of criminal justice interventions (not focussed on rehabilitation and 'cure') may be warranted or useful with such individuals (i.e., interventions that focus on addressing other factors that may in some way be associated with crime, including homelessness and poverty, past trauma and abuse, and more),[5] but at the same time, make the prospect of subjecting someone to up to two years of restricted freedoms, drug treatment and drug testing for a non-serious crime appear as an 'innovative' and 'modern' (Hulls, *Hansard,* 29 November 2001, p. 2191) solution.

Crucially, in interlocking the conceptualisations of both the 'problem' and 'solution' around bodies, control and citizenship, the addict is discursively produced as abject:[6] as *always already* criminal, and as a threat to community, public safety and more.[7] Indeed, addicts are positioned as subjects who are external to and distinct from 'the community' (and the protections typically offered to the community), precisely because their lack of control renders them a *threat* to full citizens. Such a configuration not only reinforces the dominant cultural imaginary of the addict as being a lesser citizen, but further strengthens the elevated status of the disease models of addiction (as 'disease of the will') within medicine and law, justifying an expanded role for medicine in 'curing' the addict in order to restore them to full citizenship. Thus it would seem that in the case of the Drug Court's creation, the state is willing to cede power to medicine in the pursuit of caring for the 'disordered' and 'irrational' addict – not for his or her own sake, but for the sake of others to whom they pose an unending threat.

The Assessment and Referral Court List

The Assessment and Referral Court List ('the List') was established by the *Magistrates' Court Amendment (Assessment and Referral Court List) Act 2010* (Vic). Like the Drug Court, cases heard under the List are pre-sentence, and exclude violent or sexual offences (s4S(3) *Magistrates Court Act 1989* (Vic)). Matters eligible for handling through the List must meet the following criteria:

1 *Diagnostic criteria* – the accused must be diagnosed as living with either a mental illness, intellectual disability, acquired brain injury, autism spectrum disorder, or a neurological impairment such as dementia (s4T(2) *Magistrates Court Act 1989* (Vic)).
2 *Functional criteria* – the impairment with which the accused is diagnosed must substantially reduce their capacity to undertake self-care, self-management, social interactions, or communication (s4T(3) *Magistrates Court Act 1989* (Vic)).
3 *Needs criteria* – the accused must be able to derive benefit from receiving services from an individual support plan, this includes services pertaining to disability, mental health, housing, welfare and/or health (s4T(4) *Magistrates Court Act 1989* (Vic)).

Faultless individuals suffering from a criminalising affliction

The List was debated in Victoria's Parliament in December 2009, February 2010 and March 2010. Like the Drug Court, these debates provide access to deep-seated presuppositions surrounding the purported lives of people with cognitive impairments or mental illness. In particular, members of the Legislative Assembly appear to rely on a medicalised and protectionist discourse of disability and mental health. This discourse positions cognitive impairments and mental illness as inherently negative conditions which produce lives characterised by tragedy and constant struggle, and which require intervention for the sake of 'the vulnerable' (see Oliver, 1990). In this vein, members of the Legislative Assembly present people with cognitive impairments or mental illness as 'some of the most vulnerable people in the state' (Drum, *Hansard*, 25 February 2010, p. 545), who are 'suffering' (Donnellan, *Hansard*, 3 February 2010, p. 137; Wakeling, *Hansard*, 3 February 2010, p. 138; Clark, *Hansard*, 2 February, 2010, p. 54) from a devastating 'affliction' (Drum, *Hansard*, 25 February 2010, p. 545) which is 'not the fault' of the person (Thomson, *Hansard*, 2 February 2010, p. 59), but rather a 'medical condition' (Thomson, *Hansard*, 23 March 2010, p. 937). Indeed we are told that 'people with mental illness are often the most unhappy, the most disturbed, the most troubled persons in our society, who have the greatest difficulty in dealing with day-to-day life' (Scott, *Hansard*, 2 February 2010, p. 68). What is of interest for our purposes however, is what this familiar medicalised and protectionist narrative facilitates when it appears within broader discussions of law and order; that is, its discursive, subjectification and lived effects.

By rendering people with cognitive impairments or mental illness 'faultless' victims of a debilitating 'affliction', members of the parliamentary debates give rise to the notion that crimes committed by people with cognitive impairments or mental illness are subject to the same restrictions. Indeed, members explain that many people with cognitive impairments or mental illness find themselves before the courts 'through no fault of their own' (Herbert, *Hansard*, 23 March 2010, p. 935), and that this occurs 'primarily as a consequence of their various afflictions' (Drum, *Hansard*, 25 February 2010, p. 545).

In Bacchi's sense, these passages provide access to some important, underpinning conceptual logics. There is a clear assumption that a person's cognitive impairment or mental illness somehow *creates*, or at the very least, *facilitates* criminality. Indeed, regardless of whether we are told that crime occurs because the person's 'affliction' causes them to act in ways 'they do not fully understand' (Clark, *Hansard*, 23 March 2010, p. 932), or because there are, apparently, 'parents trying to help through the system children found guilty of criminal offences when we as a community should have seen that behaviour as the workings of their medical condition' (Carli, *Hansard*, 23 March 2010, p. 937), it is a clear that criminality is understood as being linked to a person's cognitive impairment or mental illness; that it is derived from their 'medical condition'.

This is a familiar narrative as well. Mental illness in general, and schizophrenia in particular, often appear within our cultural imaginary as catalysts for uncontrolled violent behaviour (Glover-Thomas, 2011). Similarly, it is often suggested in court hearings that people with cognitive impairments are standing before the court because their impairment is simply 'unruly'

(Spivakovsky, 2014; 2015). Yet there is a slightly different representation of the 'problem' under construction here.

What is being problematised through members of the Legislative Assembly's discussion of the List is the person's agency. That is to say, it is not simply that people with cognitive impairments or mental illness are assumed to be more likely to commit a crime because of their 'affliction'; rather, their crimes occur because their 'affliction' determines all actions they take, criminal and non-criminal. The 'problem' with people with cognitive impairments or mental illness, is that they are both inherently criminal and entirely 'faultless' for being so.

This is a different construction of the 'problem' than that which underpinned the advent of Victoria's Drug Court. Indeed, even though in both cases members of the Legislative Assembly identify the 'affliction' (i.e., AOD dependence, cognitive impairment, mental illness) as the primary cause of crime, the parliamentary debates surrounding the development of these courts bring into being two very different 'afflicted' individuals. The addict has the capacity to change, but 'persists' in making poor choices. The person with the cognitive impairment or mental illness, on the other hand, neither has a choice in how they behave, nor the capacity to change; he or she is wholly controlled by their unrelenting medical condition, and for this reason, becomes 'faultless'.

The assumed presence of this different kind of 'afflicted' individual within the parliamentary debates is significant. Having been rendered both agentless and faultless by their apparent 'affliction' (as opposed to defiant or illogical, as was the 'addict'), this figure opens up the possibility that both the blame for their presence *and* the responsibility for change can be found elsewhere. Indeed we are told that:

> it is the failure of the government to invest in community-based and acute mental health services and the inability of people to get access to the mental health care that they need that is leading to such people ending up in the justice system.
>
> (Wooldridge, *Hansard*, 2 February 2010, p. 63)

It is suggested that 'if more was being done at a government level' (Duncan, *Hansard*, 3 February 2010, p. 139), people wouldn't be at 'a greater risk of falling through the cracks' (Mikakos, *Hansard*, 25 February, 2010, p. 537). Or that people with cognitive impairments or mental illness: 'require ongoing intervention to prevent [themselves] from hurting themselves or others. It is not their fault that they have these illnesses. We cannot turn our backs on them once they are out of the system' (Fyffe, *Hansard*, 2 February 2010, p. 67).

Such statements produce several effects, in Bacchi's sense. Discursively, they draw a significant distinction between the *object* responsible for people with cognitive impairments or mental illness' crimes – their 'affliction' – and the *subject* responsible for their contact with the criminal justice system – the state. Subjectively, such a distinction allows for the actual person with cognitive impairments and/or mental illness – their subjecthood and agency – to be effectively removed from the problem representation itself, relocating all of their actions, behaviours and now even responsibilities and possibilities within and between the realms of medicine and governance. This move, in turn, sets the foundations for some new material, regulatory repercussions.

A civilised response to an ongoing problem

Because the 'problem' of people with cognitive impairments or mental illness' contact with the criminal justice system lies not with the person themselves, apparently, but instead within and between their unrelenting medical condition and their history of poor governance, it is no longer conceivable to hope for 'rehabilitation' and a 'cure', nor is it logical to pursue deterrence (as it was with the more agentive 'addict'). Rather, for this problem representation, the only suitable, necessary approach would be to first assess the exact nature of the person's medical condition – to understand its propensity to 'control the body' – and to then provide 'coordinated' and extensive health and welfare services which are consistently monitored by the magistrate (i.e. 'good' governance).[8] This, it is claimed, will finally 'stabilise' the accused (Clark, *Hansard*, 2 February 2010, p. 53; Hulls, *Hansard*, 10 December 2009, p. 4604).

Conceptualising the 'solution' in this way gives foundation to a new logic about people with cognitive impairments and mental illness. This conceptualisation gives rise to the notion that people with cognitive impairments and mental illness *require ongoing government intervention* in order to live in the community, that to provide anything different to this form of intervention would 'lead to a "revolving door phenomenon" where mentally impaired defendants continue to cycle through the criminal justice system with diminishing prospects for reintegration in the community' (Hulls, *Hansard*, 10 December 2009, p. 4602). Yet this concerning regulatory repercussion is largely obscured from critique by the dominant, medicalised and protectionist discourse that underpins this problem representation. That is to say, we are reminded by former Attorney-General Hulls that 'The fairness of our system, our institutions and our democracy is measured by the manner in which we treat the most vulnerable members of our community, including mentally impaired individuals' (Hulls, *Hansard*, 10 December 2009, p. 4604).

Accordingly, it is understood that it is okay to subject people with cognitive impairments and mental illness to significant intervention and surveillance because this, we are told, is 'a civilised' way of dealing with the 'problem' (Donnellan, *Hansard*, 2 February 2010, p. 70). It protects these 'vulnerable' populations from the harshness of prison, offering them a 'more dignifying and more humane' (Hulls, *Hansard*, 10 December 2009, p. 4602) way of being treated. Indeed, the List is claimed to provide people with cognitive impairments or mental illness with the 'dignity and understanding' (Somyurek,

Hansard, 25 February 2010, p. 548) that has been absent in the past; it is both 'more humane and thoughtful' (Scott, *Hansard*, 2 February 2010, p. 68) than anything that has come before.

It is at this point that we can draw some final conclusions about the dominant cultural imaginary underpinning the development of the Drug Court and Assessment and Referral Court List in Victoria.

Conclusion

The advent of 'problem-solving courts' over the past 20 years is claimed by some to represent a significant shift in the administration of justice, offering a more 'holistic' and 'generous' approach to offenders. At a time when calls to expand such courts are on the rise, including, in the Victorian context, the Drug Court (Law Reform, Drugs and Crime Prevention Committee, 2014), we considered it important to examine the presuppositions and conceptual logics underpinning the creation of such courts, along with the effects for targeted populations.

We argued that politicians responsible for developing specialist 'problem-solving' courts rely upon a dominant cultural imaginary about agency, capacity, control and the body that draws upon and is bolstered by dominant medical discourses of addiction, disability and mental health. In parliamentary debates leading up to the establishment of these courts, key figures conceptualised people living with AOD addiction, mental illness and/or cognitive impairment as inherently criminal, through extensive and repeated discussions about the multiple ways that criminal activity was produced by their respective 'afflictions'. Importantly, however, we noticed two distinct narratives emerging in relation to agency in the context of criminal offending. In the case of people experiencing AOD dependence, the 'problem' of AOD-related offending was ultimately understood as a choice/self-induced. For people with cognitive impairments or mental illness, the problem was externalised (it was the 'fault' of their all-controlling medical condition and the state's neglect). Here, the 'addict' is simultaneously and paradoxically constituted as beholden to their affliction and yet responsible for it (and for making change). On the other hand, people living with mental illness or cognitive impairment are conceptualised as beholden to their affliction but not to blame for their predicament, nor for changing it: instead, the state is seen to have failed them through inadequate resourcing and supports. We suggest that the process of tracing how these respective 'problem' populations are constituted tells us much about how policy and lawmaking processes imagine particular subjects ('addicts', the 'disabled' and the 'mentally ill') as abnormal, fixing connections, in the process, between drugs, disability, mental illness, normalcy, crime and the state. We also argued that these conceptualisations have implications for the extent to which such subjects are viewed as citizens, and that such rationalities are often used (albeit in distinct ways) to justify seemingly novel mechanisms for the regulation, intervention and control of such populations. Although we draw no firm conclusions about the overall advantages and disadvantages of specialist court systems here, we find these processes of mutual co-constitution troubling, especially insofar as these logics appear to justify and enable long-term, intensive, medico-legal interventions into the lives of subjects that are often already marginalised and stigmatised.

We also consider it to be particularly problematic that sweeping generalisations are made about large, diverse populations of subjects such as 'the mentally ill' without proper consideration of the many differences and distinctions between people who experience mental illness. Although it may seem obvious, it is worth pointing out that people understood to be addicts, experiencing mental health issues or cognitive impairment are a heterogeneous population with diverse subjectivities, histories and motivations. In the materials we analysed here, we see a tendency in spite of this for parliamentarians to discursively produce both groups as one-dimensional, inherently dangerous and otherwise predictable cohorts with a deep-rooted propensity for criminal behaviour. In Bacchi's sense, these debates reflect the limits on what can be thought or said about these subjects, producing them instead as 'abject', abnormal, risky and *always already* a threat to society. Arguably, these processes may enhance the stigmatisation and marginalisation experienced by these populations. At the same time, other ways of thinking about the origins and solutions to crime are foreclosed, including the possibility that multiple, compounding factors contribute to their contact with criminal justice systems. In our view, there is a need for more research into how the statements of policymakers and legislators reflect dominant cultural imaginaries, shaping the ways by which 'problems' are constituted and foreclosing other possible problematisations. Future work may include an analysis of the presuppositions of vulnerability and risk that are often invoked to justify these alternative approaches to criminal justice, the effects that follow for targeted populations, and the possible benefits of alternative problematisations.

Notes

1 This chapter is derived in part from an article published in *Continuum* on 10 Feb 2017, available online: www.tandfonline.com/10.1080/10304312.2016.1275152
2 AOD is commonly used in alcohol and other drug research as a descriptor to encapsulate substances that are associated with elevated risks and harms. It is a broad and fluid category that incorporates both licit and illicit substances.
3 According to Bacchi (2009), authors should also undertake to apply the questions to their own problem representations.
4 This is not the only reference to a (imprecise and undefined) notion of the 'antisocial'. Although it is beyond the scope of this chapter to explore this issue in more depth, we note the strong normalising tendency of this descriptor. We suggest that it is important, in examining the pervasive cultural logics in these debates, to consider who gets to judge what counts as 'anti-social' and how the anti-social is

conceptualised. Conceptualisations of what is 'social' or 'anti-social' enable and sustain, among other things, particular practices of governance, with implications – material and discursive – for subjects.

5 We acknowledge that these associations are themselves contested and complex, and offer no opinion, here, on the validity of them (for more, see Seear & Fraser, 2014).

6 Here, our use of the word 'abject' is informed by the work of Judith Butler: particularly, *Bodies that Matter* (1993) and *Gender Trouble* (1990). Butler defines the 'abject' as a concept that 'relates to all kinds of bodies whose lives are not considered to be "lives" and whose materiality is understood not to "matter". To give something of an indication: the U.S. press regularly figures non-Western lives in such terms. Impoverishment is another common candidate, as is the domain of those identified as psychiatric "cases"' (Meijer & Prins, 1998, p. 281).

7 See, for example, the Hansard record (27 February 2002, p. 118), in which Wynn MP claimed that: 'The government is committed to safety on our streets, in our homes and workplaces, and has tackled the problems of drug addiction in a creative way.'

8 As Thomson explains, 'it is not about just having services there, which at the moment is the situation in most courts: an assessment of what may be needed by an individual is being made and service links are being made, but no single monitoring of the needs of that person is going on. This program will change that ...' (Thomson, *Hansard*, 2 February 2010, p. 59).

References

Australian Bureau of Statistics (ABS) (2010). *National Health Survey: Summary of Results, 2007–2008* (Reissue). Canberra: ABS.

Australian Institute of Health and Welfare (AIHW) (2011). *2010 National Drug Strategy Household Survey Report*. Drug statistics series no. 25. Cat. No. PHE 145. Canberra: AIHW.

Australian Institute of Health and Welfare (AIHW) (2012). *The Mental Health of Prison Entrants in Australia 2010*. Bulletin no. 104. Cat. No. AUS 158. Canberra: AIHW.

Australian Institute of Health and Welfare (AIHW) (2013). *The Health of Australia's Prisoners 2012*. Cat. No PHE 170. Canberra: AIHW.

Bacchi, C. (2009). *Analysing policy: what's the problem represented to be?* Sydney: Pearson Education.

Bacchi, C., & Beasley, C. (2002). Citizen bodies: Is embodies citizenship a contradiction in terms? *Critical Social Policy* 22(2), 324–352.

Bacchi, C., & Eveline, J. (2010). Approaches to gender mainstreaming: What's the problem represented to be? In C. Bacchi & J. Eveline (Eds.), *Mainstreaming politics: Gendering practices and feminist theory* (pp. 111–138). Adelaide: University of Adelaide Press.

Boldt, R. (2002). The adversary system and attorney role in the drug treatment movement. In J. Nolan (Ed.), *Drug courts in theory and practice* (pp. 115–144). New York: Aldine de Gruyter.

Boothroyd, R., Mercado, C., Poythress, N., Christy, A., & Petrilia, J. (2005) Clinical outcomes of defendants in mental health court, *Psychiatry Services* 56(7), 829–834.

Butler, J. (1993). *Bodies that matter: On the discursive limits of 'sex'*. New York: Routledge.

Butler, J. (1990). *Gender trouble: Feminism and the subversion of identity.* New York: Routledge.

Butler, T., Allnutt, S., Cain, D., Owens, D., & Muller, C. (2005). Mental disorder in the New South Wales prisoner population. *Australian and New Zealand Journal of Psychiatry* 39(5), 407–413.

Cosden, M., Ellens, J., Schnell, J., Yamini-Diouf, Y., & Wolfe, M. (2003). Evaluation of a mental health treatment court with assertive community treatment. *Behavioral Sciences and the Law* 21, 415–427.

Foucault, M. (1988). The concern for truth. Translated by A. Sheridan. In L. D. Kritzman (Ed.), *Michel Foucault: Politics, philosophy, culture: Interviews and other writings, 1977–1984* (pp. 255–267). New York: Routledge.

Fraser, S. (2004). 'It's your life!': Injecting drug users, individual responsibility and hepatitis C prevention. *Health: An Interdisciplinary Journal for the Social Study of Health, Illness and Medicine* 8(2), 199–221.

Fraser, S., & Seear, K. (2011). *Making disease, making citizens: The politics of hepatitis C.* Aldershot: Ashgate.

Glover-Thomas, N. (2011). The age of risk: Risk perception and determination following the Mental Health Act 2007. *Medical Law Review* 19, 581–605.

Hannah-Moffat, K., & Maurutto, P. (2012). Shifting and targeted forms of penal governance: Bail, punishment and specialized courts. *Theoretical Criminology* 16(2), 201–219.

Herinckz, H., Swart, S., Ama, S., Dolezal, C., & King, S. (2005). Rearrest and linkage to mental health services among clients of the Clark County Mental Health Court Program. *Psychiatry Services* 56(7), 853–857.

Keane, H. (2002). *What's wrong with addiction?* Melbourne: Melbourne University Press.

Lamberti, J., Weisman, R., Schwarzkopf, S., Price, N., Ashton, R., & Trompeter, J. (2001). The mentally ill in jails and prisons: Towards an integrated model of preventions. *Psychiatric Quarterly* 79(1), 63–77.

Lancaster, K., Seear, K., & Treloar, C. (2015). Laws prohibiting peer distribution of injecting equipment in Australia: A critical analysis of their effects. *International Journal of Drug Policy* 26(12), 1198–1206.

Law Reform, Drugs and Crime Prevention Committee (2014). *Inquiry into the Supply and Use of Methamphetamine in Victoria.* Melbourne: Parliament House.

McNeil, D., & Binder, R. (2007). Effectiveness of a mental health court in reducing criminal recidivism and violence. *American Journal of Psychiatry* 164(9), 1395–1403.

Meijer, I. C., & Prins, B. (1998). How bodies come to matter: An interview with Judith Butler. *Signs* 23(2), 275–286.

Morrell, R., Merbitz, C., & Jain, S. (1998). Traumatic brain injury in prisoners. *Journal of Offender Rehabilitation* 27, 1–8.

Moore, D. (2007). Translating justice and therapy: The Drug Treatment Court networks. *British Journal of Criminology* 47(1), 42–60.

Oliver, M. (1990). *The politics of disablement.* Basingstoke: Macmillian and St Martin's Press.

Prins, S. (2011). Does transinstitutionalisation explain the overrepresentation of people with serious mental illness in the criminal justice system? *Community Mental Health Journal* 47, 716–722.

Schofield, P., Butler, T., & Hollis, S. (2007). *October 2007 Forum – Injury Control Council of Western Australia. Hunder Forensic Head Injury Project*. Perth: National Drug Research Institute.

Seear, K., & Fraser, S. (2014). The addict as victim: Producing the 'problem' of addiction in Australian victims of crime compensation laws. *International Journal of Drug Policy* 25(5), 826–835.

Spivakovsky, C. (2014). From punishment to protection: Containing and controlling the lives of people with disabilities in human rights. *Punishment & Society* 16(5), 560–577.

Spivakovsky, C. (2015). Making dangerousness intelligible in intellectual disability. *Griffith Law Review* 23(3), 389–404.

Steadman, H., Redlich, A., Callahan, L., Robbins, P., & Vesselinov, R. (2011). Effect of mental health courts on arrests and jail days: A multisite study. *Arch Gen Psychiatry* 68(2), 167–172.

Wexler, D., & Winick, B. (Eds.) (1996). *Law in a therapeutic key: Therapeutic jurisprudence and the courts*. Durham: Carolina Academic Press.

Legislation and parliamentary debates

Magistrates' Court Act 1989 (Vic)

Magistrates' Court Amendment (Assessment and Referral Court List) Act 2010 (Vic)

Parliament of Victoria, Legislative Assembly, Parliamentary Debates, Thursday, 10 December 2009. www.parliament.vic.gov.au/hansard

Parliament of Victoria, Legislative Assembly, Parliamentary Debates, Tuesday, 2 February 2010. www.parliament.vic.gov.au/hansard

Parliament of Victoria, Legislative Assembly, Parliamentary Debates, Wednesday, 3 February 2010. www.parliament.vic.gov.au/hansard

Parliament of Victoria, Legislative Council, Parliamentary Debates, Thursday, 25 February 2010. www.parliament.vic.gov.au/hansard

Parliament of Victoria, Legislative Assembly, Parliamentary Debates, Tuesday, 23 March 2010. www.parliament.vic.gov.au/hansard

Sentencing Act 1991 (Vic)

Sentencing (Amendment) Act 2002 (Vic)

Chapter 8

The Healthy Welfare Card

Indigenous empowerment or 'remote control'?

Stephen Gray

In March 2016, the first trial of potentially the most radical reform to Australia's social security system in decades, the Healthy Welfare Card, began in Ceduna, South Australia (Teece-Johnson, 2016). In late April, trials began in the second of three envisaged sites, communities in and around Kununurra in Western Australia (WA)'s East Kimberley region. The third site has yet to be publicly identified, although discussion has centred around the goldfields area of regional WA (Martin, 2016). Trials will last for 12 months in each location, involving up to 10,000 participants at any particular time. They are scheduled to conclude by 30 June 2018 (Commonwealth of Australia, 2015).

The Healthy Welfare Card was a key recommendation of Australian mining magnate Andrew Forrest's review of Indigenous jobs and training, *Creating Parity – the Forrest Review*, commissioned by the federal government in 2014 (Forrest, 2014). Now enshrined in the *Social Security Legislation Amendment (Debit Card Trial) Bill* 2015, the card is designed 'to test the concept of cashless welfare arrangements by disbursing particular welfare payments to a restricted bank account, accessed by a debit card which does not allow cash withdrawals' (Commonwealth of Australia, 2015). A default amount of 80% of a trial participant's welfare payments is placed into such an account.

The card is intended to 'work as similarly as possible to any other bank card,' and to work at 'all existing terminals and shops, except those exclusively selling restricted products' such as alcohol and gambling products or cash withdrawals (Commonwealth of Australia, 2015, p. 1). While the Forrest Review recommended that all of a recipient's welfare payment go into such an account (Forrest, 2014, p. 104), the trial has accepted that 'people need cash for minor expenses such as children's lunch money or bus fares'. Consequently it allowed the remaining 20% of welfare payments to be available in cash.

Trial participants are determined 'based upon a combination of class of person, receipt of particular welfare payments, known as trigger payments, and particular trial areas' (Commonwealth of Australia, 2015, p. 4). A legislative instrument may determine that a particular trigger payment applies in relation to a trial area. Trigger payments include all the major social security benefits available to people of working age, including Newstart (unemployment benefit) and Youth Allowance (broadly, student or training payments), carer payment and disability support payment. A 'community body' may be authorised under section 124PE of the Bill, with that body able to reach agreements with individual trial participants varying the amount of that person's social security benefit made subject to the scheme, as long as the restricted portion is not less than 50% and not more than 80% of the total payment. The government has so far sought agreement with relevant community bodies before proceeding with the trial.

It is a striking feature of the Healthy Welfare Card that the vast majority of the people subject to the trials are Indigenous. This includes nearly all trial participants in the East Kimberley, and over 70% in Ceduna (see, e.g., Altman, 2016), both Ceduna and the Kimberley being parts of Australia with high Indigenous populations. If the third trial site is in regional WA as appears currently envisaged, most participants in that trial as well are likely to be Aboriginal.

This chapter will argue that the Healthy Welfare Card is a continuation of white Australia's historic efforts at coercive assimilation of Indigenous people into the mainstream. The introduction of the Card is ideologically driven, predicated on a notion of the deserving welfare recipient which is entirely inconsistent with Indigenous culture. The language used by the Card's proponents is also disturbingly at odds with the reality of its operation. While ostensibly the Card is designed to empower its recipients to participate in the mainstream economy and hence lead 'healthy' and 'meaningful' lives, its effect is likely to be a further stigmatising of Indigenous welfare recipients and the instigation of further resistance to the Card.

The first part of the chapter will briefly outline the main features of white Australian attempts at controlling Indigenous access to cash, whether in the form of wages or of social security. The second part will consider the Northern Territory's income management regime (IMR), part of the Northern Territory Intervention which began in 2007, and a recent attempt to regulate Indigenous economic participation with significant similarities to the Healthy Welfare Card. The third and fourth parts of the chapter will move to a closer consideration of the language and operation of the Card. They will consider the slippage in the language of the Card's proponents on the question of whether its true target is social security recipients in general, or Aboriginal people in particular. The fifth section of the chapter will consider the extent to which these factors are likely to engender Indigenous resistance, as has occurred with similar programs in the past. Finally, the chapter will suggest how the Card might be reformulated in order to avoid what otherwise seems its inevitable failure to achieve its stated aims.

A historical sketch: White Australia's attempts to control indigenous access to cash

From Australia's early colonial period, Indigenous people were regarded as incapable of handling cash (see Bielefeld, 2014b, p. 99). On the missions and pastoral leases of the colonial frontier, Aboriginal people were kept in slave-like conditions, with variable numbers employed depending on seasonal needs, and payments made 'in kind'. In this environment, even the protectors charged with looking after the interests of Aboriginal people considered that cash wages would have only a degrading and demoralising effect. The celebrated anthropologist Professor Baldwin Spencer, for example, as Chief Protector of Aborigines in the Northern Territory (NT) in 1912, thought that cash wages would turn the Aboriginal worker from being a 'cheerful worker and perfectly happy' to a 'useless loafer', the 'so-called civilised native in the settlement, who has learned the value of money because it buys him clothing and opium' (Gray, 2011, p. 47).

As a consequence, 'protective' legislation either required payment of wages at rates far less than those applicable to European employees, or did not require cash wages at all. Even where wages were theoretically payable, the laws were not enforced. In the 1920s, for example, agricultural workers at Daly River 'were lucky if they got a clay pipe and a stick of tobacco when the year's work was done. They were fed ... mainly on cobs or corn with an occasional handful or two of peanuts' (Gray, 2011, p. 54).

When Aboriginal people did receive wages, the money was frequently held in Aboriginal trust accounts. Again, this was ostensibly for their benefit, so that they might be taught habits of thrift, and their wages spent on worthwhile goals such as housing. However, these trust accounts were frequently abused, especially in Queensland, where 'the state frequently raided... [them] in order to finance the reserve and mission system that incarcerated Indigenous peoples' (Bielefeld, 2014b, p. 102). In the last 15 years, public awareness of this issue has increased, leading to the establishment of trust fund repayment schemes in several Australian states, although not in the NT (Gray, 2007, 2008; Thornton & Luker, 2009). Needless to say, the adequacy of repayment schemes has also been much criticised (see, e.g., Anthony, 2013).

Far less generally known is the history of Indigenous people's dealing with Australia's social security system. 'Aboriginal natives' were excluded from Australia's first federal social security legislation, the *Invalid and Old-Age Pensioners Act 1908* (Cth), and the *Maternity Allowance Act 1912* (Cth), along with 'Asiatics' and other 'coloured' groups (see Gray, 2011; Kewley, 1973). Social security benefits were first payable to 'aboriginal natives' under the *Child Endowment Act 1941* (Cth). With the coming of the assimilation era, the *Social Services Act 1959* (Cth) repealed those parts of previous legislation which had allowed benefits to be paid only to 'exempt' Aboriginal people. However, general provisions continued to allow the Department of

Social Services to pay pensions and allowances directly to missions, pastoral lessees or other institutions.

Thus, child endowment was normally paid direct to the missions or pastoral leases on which many Aboriginal people lived. It was almost impossible for officials to keep track of the numbers of children entitled to endowment, and of the movement of children in family groups from one place to another. This made it easy for pastoralists to claim endowment in respect of more children than were actually maintained. In addition, there was no way for the Welfare Branch to keep track of whether pastoralists actually spent welfare money on the upkeep of the child. The same applied to missions, who could claim money in respect of children who did not actually live on the mission all year round. Again, missions were not required in practice to spend endowment money on the child; they could use it to build schools, hospitals and clinics, as well as 'training centres' for arts and crafts (see Gray, 2011, pp. 140–1).

Similar practices existed in relation to unemployment and sickness benefits, and aged and invalid pensions. In 1963 on one Territory community, the aged pension was paid direct to the mission, which used it to build houses, toilets, shower blocks and water reticulation, a practice condoned by the Department of Social Services. This meant that missions were officially permitted to use pensioners' money to provide basic services which 'would have been taken for granted in the towns' (Gray, 2011, p. 139).

Given the long history of official withholding and misappropriation of money owed to Indigenous people, it is not surprising that such people might view bureaucratic assertions of the need to withhold pensions and allowances for the recipient's own good with suspicion. This distrust was particularly evident in the more recent reaction to the NT's IMR.

Regulating the Indigenous economy: the Northern Territory's income management regime

The IMR was introduced in 2007 as part of the Northern Territory Intervention, then known as the Emergency Response. It formed part of the Commonwealth government's response to the *Little Children Are Sacred* inquiry into allegations of sexual abuse of children on Aboriginal communities (see Northern Territory Government, 2007; Parliamentary Joint Committee on Human Rights, 2016). Even at the time, the link between sexual abuse and income management was somewhat tenuous, resting on an assertion from 'some people' who gave evidence to the inquiry that if welfare was quarantined it might impact positively on alcohol consumption, and hence, presumably, on sexual abuse. The inquiry's tentative suggestion that income management was 'worth investigating' was taken up in spades by the Howard government, which introduced its management scheme to the vast majority of Indigenous people in the Territory on income support.

In its original form, income management applied to 73 prescribed communities, and 10 town camp regions in the NT. It quarantined 50% of a welfare recipient's income, which could only be spent using a government-issued card (known as a BasicsCard) with a personal identification number (Bielefeld, 2014a, p. 696). Income-managed funds could only be spent in certain stores, and could not be used to purchase excluded items such as alcohol, tobacco or pornography, or be used for gambling.

As it effectively applied only to Aboriginal people, the IMR in its original form required the suspension of the *Racial Discrimination Act* (1975). The incoming Rudd Labor Government promised to reinstate the Act in its application to the NT Emergency Response. In 2010 it did so, passing legislation to extend income management to all welfare recipients in the NT, provided they met certain criteria (*Social Security and Other Legislation Amendment (Welfare Reform and Reinstatement of the Racial Discrimination Act) Act 2010;* Parliamentary Joint Committee on Human Rights, 2016, p. 37). The regime was modified again by the Stronger Futures package of legislation in 2012, enabling a range of state and territory authorities to refer locations outside the NT for income management. Thus in 2016, it applied to 15 locations outside the NT (Parliamentary Joint Committee on Human Rights, 2016, p. 38).

By 2013, a person in the NT could be subjected to compulsory income management if they were classed as a 'long-term welfare payment recipient' (aged over 25, and in receipt of unemployment benefits, youth allowance or parenting payments for 12 of the last 24 months); disengaged youth (aged 15 to 24, and receiving youth allowance, unemployment benefits or parenting payments for three of the last six months); or 'vulnerable income management referrals' (on most welfare benefits, and referred for income management by a Centrelink social worker, a child protection worker, or by the Territory's Alcohol Mandatory Treatment Tribunal) (Parliamentary Joint Committee on Human Rights, 2016, p. 38). There is also a category of 'voluntary' income management. Income-managed funds might be subject to automatic deductions to meet a range of 'priority needs' such as food and rent, with the remainder still only accessible using the BasicsCard (Parliamentary Joint Committee on Human Rights, 2016, p. 39).

Not unexpectedly, the IMR has been extensively criticised. Mendes (2013) argues that it represents a 'fundamental shift in Australian income security policy from structural to individualistic explanations of social disadvantage' (pp. 493, 495). It views people as being on welfare not because of the economy, but because they are lazy, or immoral, or incompetent. Bielefeld (2014a) argues that the law 'constructs, rather than merely describes, the vulnerability that the Government claims to seek to redress via these laws' (p. 699). She questions the process through which Centrelink (broadly, social security departmental) staff classify people as vulnerable, arguing that it reflects neo-liberal values in which people are individualistic, rational, acquisitive and keen to maximise their own welfare (Bielefeld, 2014a). These values are, of course, antithetical to those of Aboriginal culture, and hence represent an assimilationist agenda, designed to force Aboriginal people into the mainstream. One clear example (particularly, until 2010) is that the IMR may represent a significant practical barrier to Indigenous people moving back to the country, since if they do, they fear being subjected to the IMR.

Not all social welfare recipients are automatically subjected to income management. People on disability support payments, for example, are subjected to the regime only if they are classified as 'vulnerable' – for example, because they have been recently released from gaol, have been regarded as demonstrating budgetary incompetence, have failed to undertake reasonable self-care, or are homeless or at risk of homelessness (Bielefeld, 2014a, p. 715). However, Bielefeld cites data from 2012 showing that 77% of people classified as 'vulnerable welfare recipients' received a Disability Support Pension (Bielefeld, 2014a, p. 716). When added to the fact that on the same set of figures from 2012, 96% of those on Vulnerable Income Management were Indigenous, this raises the spectre of disability as well as racial discrimination, as Bielefeld points out (Bielefeld, 2014a, pp. 715–6; see also figures cited in Parliamentary Joint Committee on Human Rights, 2016, p. 45).

The 2016 Parliamentary Joint Committee on Human Rights uses more cautious language to raise similar concerns. It notes the government's argument that income management is not discriminatory because it is not explicitly racially based. In order for this argument to be acceptable in international law, it notes, the 'income management measures will need to be shown to be based on objective and reasonable grounds and be a proportionate measure in pursuit of a legitimate objective' (Parliamentary Joint Committee on Human Rights, 2016, p. 46). The Committee accepted that supporting 'vulnerable' welfare recipients was a rational and worthwhile objective. However, it questioned whether the IMR was 'likely to be effective in achieving the aim of supporting budgeting skills and financial acumen' (Parliamentary Joint Committee on Human Rights, 2016, p. 49). An evaluation report in September 2014 found 'no evidence that income management has achieved its intended outcomes' (The Social Policy Research Centre at the University of New South Wales (UNSW) and the Australian National University (ANU), in Parliamentary Joint Committee on Human Rights, 2016, p. 50). There was no substantive evidence that the program had changed people's behaviour, and a substantial group of people 'felt that income management is unfair, embarrassing and discriminatory' (The Social Policy Research Centre at UNSW and ANU, in Parliamentary Joint Committee on Human Rights, 2016, p. 51).

On this evidence, there seems to be a clear disconnect between the benign language of bureaucratese and the perceptions and lived experience of those Indigenous people subject to the IMR. As will become clear in the following sections, the Healthy Welfare Card raises very similar concerns.

The ideological origins of the Healthy Welfare Card: who are its true targets?

There is currently a considerable, not to say unsettling, lack of clarity concerning the true aim of the Healthy Welfare Card – whether it is aimed ultimately at all social security recipients, reconstituted as supplicants on government rather than individuals with rights, or only at Indigenous people, reconstructed in official language as the most 'vulnerable'. At first sight, the Card's origins in the Forrest Review of (specifically) Indigenous jobs and training suggests it is aimed only at Indigenous people. However, the language of that review betrays a strong ideological enthusiasm for extending the Healthy Welfare Card Australia-wide. The Review's arguments to this effect are vehement, if a little logically unclear. It argues strongly that cash payments are dangerous for vulnerable welfare recipients:

> Community leaders told us how unscrupulous commerce and organised crime have taken advantage of the cash available to vulnerable welfare recipients by specifically targeting those communities where people are at the highest risk of making poor, short-term purchase decisions, such as gambling and buying illicit drugs (like marijuana) and alcohol … First Australian Elders told us they gravely fear for their children as harder drugs such as methamphetamines with higher cash margins are now entering their communities through organised crime. These crime syndicates then target the users of marijuana, common in many remote and urban communities, with even more dangerous illicit drugs.
>
> (Forrest, 2014, pp. 102–3)

This might suggest that cashless welfare should be directed at only the 'vulnerable', particularly those whom experience has shown are addicted to alcohol or other drugs. However, the Review's arguments go much further than this. It notes that social welfare was always intended to be 'a safety net for families and individuals who need help on a temporary basis'; it should never be 'a destination of choice' (Forrest, 2014, p. 101. In place of the host of evils to which cash payments lead, the Review argues that a 'new solution [is] needed to make transitioning off welfare and into work an empowering experience so individuals can manage their financial affairs' (Forrest, 2014, p. 104).

In reaching this conclusion, the Review was 'influenced by the pioneering experience of the current income management system and BasicsCard in the Northern Territory' (Forrest, 2014, p. 104), as well as South Africa's cashless card system, introduced in 2012. It consulted with large corporations and the major banks, and noted the potential of the system not only to eradicate welfare fraud, but save 'a fortune in welfare administration' (Forrest, 2014, p. 104). So empowering would the cashless welfare system be for those subject to it, the review concludes, that 'it will render the cash system that preceded it an irresponsible social experiment' (Forrest, 2014, p. 104).

Despite its use of the language of 'empowerment', it seems clear that the Welfare Card is ideologically driven. It constructs all social welfare recipients – including, for example, those on carer or disability support payments – as incapable of managing their own financial affairs. At the same time these individuals are constructed as capable of working, and social security benefits as a mere temporary support in the journey back to the workforce. Lack of skills or education, lack of employment opportunities, and long-term disabilities or carer responsibilities are all ignored in this analysis.

Such concerns are clearly not limited to Indigenous social welfare recipients. Non-Indigenous recipients are also likely to resent this labelling, and are generally more likely to have access to media to publicise their objections, as was seen in recent controversy surrounding the introduction of income management in Western Sydney. No doubt recognising this, then Social Services Minister Scott Morrison said in March 2015 that there was:

> no suggestion at this stage that the card will have mainstream application. It's there as a key tool to target particular areas of disadvantage and to see whether it can make the big difference that we believe and hope that it can.
>
> (McDonald, 2015)

Although at time of writing the trial had barely commenced, there have already been significant expressions of concern from Indigenous people. Moree in NSW withdrew as a trial candidate site, and in Ceduna there was opposition from Aboriginal elders, who claimed there had been a 'complete lack of consultation with community members. They have only spoken to service providers, and people who work for them, not the people who will be put on the card' (see Teece-Johnson, 2016). In the Kimberley, Indigenous opinion is sharply divided, with Kununurra and Wyndham confirmed trial sites, while Hall's Creek and other outstations have declined to participate. Nevertheless, at this stage, it appears that the only people targeted are those in 'particular areas of disadvantage', or the 'vulnerable' – code, a cynic might suggest, for Indigenous people in remote areas whose protests are unlikely to garner mainstream community support.

The Healthy Welfare Card: practical concerns

Concerns have also been expressed about how the Card would operate in practice. Trial participants – that is, Indigenous welfare recipients – have complained of a complete lack of information about the Card. Details of which businesses are excluded from the Card's operation are also not included in the Bill or its explanatory memorandum, with these details being left to 'a future legislative instrument,' according to the Parliamentary Joint Committee on Human Rights (2015, p. 20).

While it seems obvious that the intention is to exclude bottle shops, it was not clear how this would work for retailers (including supermarkets) who sell a mixed range of goods such as vegetables and alcohol. According to Nicolas Rothwell (2016), the Card can still be used to buy both tobacco products, 'the chief cause of chronic disease and debility in the remote Aboriginal world', as well as pornography. On the other hand, Indigenous trial participants said that they were unclear whether the Card would be able to be used for larger purchases, such as whitegoods (fridges, ovens and similar items) or tyres. At the time of writing, it was also not clear whether the Card could be used to buy air or bus fares – for example, to travel to urban centres so that children may attend or participate in sporting events.

Cash is still used for many transactions, including markets and public transport, as well as some second-hand stores (Rothwell, 2016) – particularly in the bush, where the trials are taking place. Perhaps most importantly, the Card has significant and poorly understood impacts upon customary Indigenous methods of handling money. As Rod Hagen pointed out:

> Welfare cards assume that all transactions within Aboriginal communities occur between Aboriginal people and external vendors or service suppliers. They make no provision for exchange within the extremely important internal economy of such communities ... Even on a day to day level the direct transfer of cash between community members helps to 'even out' the huge problems faced by impoverished people. Payment of a fine, for example, may be impossible for any individual in a community but attainable by people combining their financial resources. Non-payment if such pooling is prevented by an absence of cash may result in the incarceration of a valued community member.
>
> (comment on Fletcher, 2015)

Customary 'transfer of cash' between community members has many aspects. Not only are social security moneys pooled, but people with jobs or more lucrative sources of income are obliged in various ways to pay relations without such sources. This was evident even in the 1950s, when the artist Albert Namatjira was convicted and jailed for buying alcohol for dependent relatives, then known as 'wards' (see *Namatjira v Raabe* in Gray, 2011, p. 154); it is even more relevant today, when relatives are in danger of 'being forced to surrender their money to the youthful armies of drug-using shakedown operators who maraud through communities and town camps' (Rothwell, 2016). Taken to its conclusion, the logical driver of the Healthy Welfare Card – taking away access to cash from those who might misuse it – would suggest that all Indigenous people should be deprived of such access, whether they have jobs or not. As Rothwell points out, with tongue in cheek:

No big-name indigenous artist could be paid in standard fashion, none of the salaried local staff could be left free of restrictions on their earned income, none of the vast royalty payments that form so large a part of remote area wealth could be exempt from controls.

(Rothwell, 2016)

Given these not entirely fanciful possibilities, the idea that Indigenous people might be 'empowered' by having their money taken away might sound almost like a piece of Orwellian doublespeak. This is particularly so when the lived experience of the Card's administration is one of lack of information, official confusion and, on occasions, humiliation. The following section will expand on these concerns, as well as on the Indigenous strategy of 'passive resistance' to bureaucratic authority they engender.

Passive resistance, non-compliance and bureaucratic decline

In the field of Indigenous health, well-intentioned doctors and health professionals have sometimes wondered why so many Indigenous people continue to make poor 'lifestyle choices' such as smoking or excessive drinking – or indeed why they may simply not take prescribed medication, or make changes in behaviour when the consequences of failing to follow the professional's recommendations are painstakingly described. Occasionally, such choices are ascribed partly to a strategy of non-compliance, a form of resistance to white authority which manifests itself passively, and by a strategy that looks objectively like self-harm (Kerridge, Lowe & Stewart, 2013). In the context of income management, Shelley Bielefeld has expanded upon this narrative of Indigenous passive resistance to, or non-compliance with, ostensibly well-intentioned government strategies of control. She refers to the large number of BasicsCards being replaced or 'lost' by their recipients. Indigenous people 'lose' their cards far more frequently than non-Indigenous welfare recipients: on average, during the period covered in one survey, Indigenous people had an average of 3.8 BasicsCards issued, compared to an average of 1.3 for non-Indigenous people (Bielefeld, 2014a). Interviews with recipients suggest various reasons for these 'losses' – not just itinerant lifestyles, but also cultural practices of card sharing, as well as people harassing or 'humbugging' others for their cards.

In part, these attitudes flow from the very obvious stigma associated with the NT's BasicsCard. A Centrelink officer gave the example of a sales assistant in a supermarket who told the customer she could not have the more expensive steak, but had to 'go and get that other steak, that cheaper one,' because they were 'on that card' (Bielefeld, 2014a, p. 720). During consultations, Aboriginal people expressed anger and frustration at this kind of treatment while using the BasicsCard. BasicsCard users reported being told by shop assistants that their choice of purchases was inappropriate. They felt stigmatised as 'deficient' or as 'bad mothers,' and felt that going to the supermarket was a 'shame job,' forcing them to shop in a supermarket away from their home to avoid being seen using the card (The Social Policy Research Centre at UNSW and ANU 2012, cited in Parliamentary Joint Committee on Human Rights, 2016, pp. 57–58). It seems clear that a card designed in theory to empower Indigenous people in fact has the practical effect of reconstituting them as vulnerable, as incapable of managing their own money.

It is clear that this strategy of passive non-compliance is a pervasive response in Indigenous communities, particularly in remote areas, and that it is directed generally at official interventions, not just at income management. Nicolas Rothwell has analysed this strategy in the context of a general question that:

> no one in the circles of administrative power wants to ask clearly, or answer squarely: why aren't the men and women of Indigenous communities across the deserts and the north sending their children to school, seeking out jobs and training opportunities, engaging with the scores of programs under way in their midst?
>
> (Rothwell, 2015)

Rothwell's answer is entirely consistent with Bielefeld's, and indeed with many decades of post-colonial analysis: resistance. Resistance is a historical feature of Indigenous response to colonialism. However, as Rothwell (2015) points out, resistance is especially strong to the new (and bipartisan) 'ruling paradigm' in Indigenous affairs, close surveillance and control of community affairs backed by penalty and incentive, or more simply the carrot and the stick. Resistance exists regardless of whether the system is well-intentioned, its goal to 'cut into welfare dependency while senior community members who remembered another system were still living' (Rothwell, 2015) or whether more sinister motives were intermingled, in particular the goal of undermining the power of Aboriginal land councils and gaining 'easy access to indigenous land'. The reasons for resistance have deep roots in history: the identity of Indigenous Australians as a 'dispossessed people, conscious their world is occupied by outsiders' (Rothwell, 2015).

One facet of this resistance is two 'quite separate modes of expression: one for when white people are around, one for themselves' (Rothwell, 2015). When 'consulted', Indigenous people may express their desire to work in mainstream jobs, or send their children to school, or stop drinking or smoking; but their behaviour in reality expresses the opposite desire. This may be particularly true of very remote communities, whose people have in fact little genuine interest in mainstream social norms such as school attendance, work and home ownership. Within this strategy 'self-neglect, poor health and social harm are also expressions of ... the veto Aborigines hold in their hands over

Australian society and its representatives' (Rothwell, 2015). The more strictly or stringently government tries to impose mainstream norms upon bush communities, the greater the level of resistance.

Such an analysis presents an admittedly rather depressing view of the capacity of any government program to affect Indigenous lives in some positive way. To a pessimist, this would seem to be as true of programs informed by 'consultation' and inspired by ideals of self-determination as of top-down, command and control interventions – since any consultation is almost by definition not real, and the notion of self-determination a chimera for people whose capacity to control their own lives was wrestled from them generations ago. However, this analysis underlines the overarching need for programs to be driven – and, preferably, led – by the Indigenous communities for whose benefit they are intended. This is as true of the Healthy Welfare Card as of income management, school attendance, family violence programs or any other of the original Northern Territory Intervention's initiatives.

Conclusion – programs driven by community need?

In March 2016, the Parliamentary Joint Committee on Human Rights made two significant recommendations in relation to the NT's IMR. Firstly, it recommended that community-led income management only occur 'where there has been a formal request for income management in a particular community following effective consultation on the particular modalities of its operation, including whether it should be a voluntary program' (Parliamentary Joint Committee on Human Rights, 2016, p. 62). In other words, income management in a community must be driven by that community. Secondly, it recommended that income management only be imposed on a person 'when that person has been individually assessed as not able to appropriately manage their income support payments. Information concerning rights and processes of appeal should be provided to the person immediately and in a language that they understand' (Parliamentary Joint Committee on Human Rights, 2016, p. 62).

These observations are as true of the Healthy Welfare Card as of income management. In fact, it may be said that they are more true, since the Healthy Welfare Card is more interventionist and draconian in several ways – in particular, because it sequesters a greater percentage of income than does income management, and because it applies compulsorily to a greater range of 'trigger payments' than income management, including, for example, the disability support pension. In any case, the experience of income management, as well as many decades of government control of indigenous people's income during the pre-Whitlam years, suggests overwhelmingly that such measures only have a chance of success if driven by, and not imposed upon, Aboriginal people.

By no means can the same be said of the current trials of the Healthy Welfare Card. Rather, as this chapter has argued, the Healthy Welfare Card is likely to be seen as yet another example of a longstanding white Australian project, the attempt to command and control Indigenous wages and spending, with an ultimately assimilationist aim. Given this reality, the Card is unlikely to succeed unless it is reformulated in a way that is community driven and designed to suit community needs. In its current form, as this chapter has argued, the Card embodies a paradox, or a form of doublespeak. It purports to enable its recipients to participate in the mainstream economy while restricting their ability to do so: in other words, disempowering in order to empower.

References

Altman, J. (2016, February 25). *Will the healthy welfare card be healthy?* School of Regulation and Global Governance, Australian National University. http://regnet. anu.edu.au/news-events/news/6371/will-healthy-welfare-card-be-healthy

Anthony, T. (2013). Indigenous stolen wages: Historical exploitation and contemporary injustice. *Precedent* 118, 42–46.

Bielefeld, S. (2014a). Compulsory income management and indigenous peoples – exploring counter narratives amidst colonial constructions of vulnerability. *Sydney Law Review* 36, 695–726.

Bielefeld, S. (2014b). Compulsory income management, Indigenous peoples and structural violence – implications for citizenship and autonomy. *Australian Indigenous Law Report* 18(1), 99–118.

Commonwealth of Australia (2015). *Explanatory Memorandum, Social Security Legislation Amendment (Debit Card Trial) Bill 2015.*

Fletcher, A. (2015, October 6). Andrew Forrest's Healthy Welfare Card – a Basicscard with added human rights? *The Castan Centre Human Rights Blog.* https://casta ncentre.com/2015/10/06/andrew-forrests-healthy-welfare-card-a-basicscard-with-added-h uman-rights/

Forrest, A. (2014). *Creating parity – the Forrest Review.* Department of Prime Minister and Cabinet. http://indigenousjobsandtrainingreview.dpmc.gov.au/

Gray, S. (2007). The elephant in the drawing room: Slavery and the 'stolen wages' debate. *Australian Indigenous Law Review* 1(1), 30–53.

Gray, S. (2008). Holding the government to account: The 'stolen wages' issue, fiduciary duty and trust. *Melbourne University Law Review* 32(1), 115–140.

Gray, S. (2011). *Brass discs, dog tags and finger scanners: The apology and Aboriginal protection in the Northern Territory 1863–1972.* Darwin: Charles Darwin University Press.

Kerridge, I., Lowe, M., & Stewart, C. (2013). *Ethics and law for the health professions* (4th ed). Annandale: Federation Press.

Kewley, T. H. (1973). *Social security in Australia 1900–1972.* Sydney: Sydney University Press.

Martin, S. (2016, January 20). National cashless welfare card plan by Turnbull government. *The Australian.* www.theaustralian.com.au/national-affairs/national-ca

shless-welfare-card-plan-by-turnbull-government/news-story/097dfa3a1bfc867afa5f8
b298c43c248

McDonald, S. (2015, March 23). Federal government to trial cashless welfare card,
with payments not allowed to be spent on alcohol or gambling. *ABC News*. www.
abc.net.au/news/2015-03-22/government-trial-cashless-welfare-card-payments-alcohol-
gambling/6339080

Mendes, P. (2013). Compulsory income management: A critical examination of the
emergence of conditional welfare in Australia. *Australian Social Work* 66(4), 495–510.

Northern Territory Government (2007). *Report of the Northern Territory Board of
Inquiry into the Protection of Aboriginal Children from Sexual Abuse; Ampe Ake-
lyernemane Meke Mekarle: Little Children are Sacred*. Darwin: Northern Territory
Government.

Parliamentary Joint Committee on Human Rights (2015). *Human Rights Scrutiny
Report*. Canberra: Commonwealth of Australia.

Parliamentary Joint Committee on Human Rights (2016). *2016 Review of Stronger
Futures Measures*. Canberra: Commonwealth of Australia.

Rothwell, N. (2015, January 24). Rebellion thwarts remote control. *The Australian*.
www.theaustralian.com.au/national-affairs/indigenous/rebellion-thwarts-remote-con
trol/news-story/4735bbc3e9c107461c804b3bc214f9ef

Rothwell, N. (2016, February 20). Cashless welfare card draws on bankrupt indigenous policy. *The Australian*. www.theaustralian.com.au/news/inquirer/cashless-welfa
re-card-for-draws-on-bankrupt-indigenous-policy/news-story/51ef26ef32aadfc1e7411
c0adda1084f

Teece-Johnson, D. (2016, March 15). On the ground in Ceduna on day one of the
Healthy Welfare Card trial. *The Point*. www.sbs.com.au/nitv/the-point-with-stan-gra
nt/article/2016/03/15/ground-ceduna-day-one-healthy-welfare-card-trial

Thornton, M., & Luker, T. (2009). The wages of sin: Compensation for Indigenous
workers. *UNSW Law Journal* 32(3), 647–673.

Legislation

Child Endowment Act 1941 (Cth)
Invalid and Old-Age Pensioners Act 1908 (Cth)
Maternity Allowance Act 1912 (Cth)
*Social Security and Other Legislation Amendment (Welfare Reform and Reinstatement
of the Racial Discrimination Act) Act 2010* (Cth)
Social Services Act 1959 (Cth)

Cases

Namatjira v Raabe (1958) NTJ 608

Chapter 9

Sterilisation, disability and well-being

The curative imaginary of the 'welfare jurisdiction'

Linda Steele

The Family Court of Australia (FCA), operating in its 'welfare jurisdiction', can authorise parental consent to sterilisation of children with intellectual disability ('court-authorised sterilisation') where the sterilisation is in the 'best interests' of the child and there are no less invasive alternatives. While legally capable of being ordered in relation to girls and boys, sterilisation is overwhelmingly a gendered phenomenon applicable to girls. When court authorisation was first established as necessary by the High Court of Australia (HCA) in *Secretary, Department of Health and Community Services v JWB* (1992) 175 CLR 218 (*Marion's Case*), this approach was viewed as protective because it provided oversight to parental decisions. Yet, this approach actually set up a system of 'protective' *regulation* of sterilisation but now with greater state complicity in the process, rather than an alternative approach of *prohibiting* sterilisation outright. As such, since at least the 1980s, court-authorised sterilisation has had a politically and ethically contentious status in Australian law, as evidenced by the number of law reform reports on this issue (Senate Community Affairs References Committee, 2013, pp. 2–4) and the consistent criticism by disability rights activists of sterilisation as a state sanctioned mode of discrimination, violence and torture (Frohmader, 2013). Since the coming into force in 2008 of the United Nations *Convention on the Rights of Persons with Disabilities* (CRPD), these disability rights criticisms have intensified and been supported by United Nations condemnation of Australia's regulatory approach to sterilisation. Yet, court-authorised sterilisation remains lawful in Australia. Indeed, as recently as 2013, the Senate Community Affairs Reference Committee affirmed the important role of the FCA in this practice (Senate Community Affairs References Committee, 2013).

In earlier scholarship, I have analysed court-authorised sterilisation as lawful violence, drawing attention to the complicity of law and the state in this violence (Steele, 2014; 2016). Building on this scholarship and of particular relevance to this edited collection's focus on *court-mandated* interventions, in this chapter I focus on how the judiciary, as one arm of state authority (the other two being the executive and legislature), is positioned to legitimately authorise the violence of sterilisation. I do this through an examination of the FCA's jurisdiction to authorise sterilisation, because jurisdiction refers to the court's 'authority to decide' (*Minister for Immigration, Migration and Indigenous Affairs v B* (2004) 219 CLR 365 (*MIMIA v B*), 377 [6]). In being a federal court, the FCA's jurisdiction is not only constrained by its constitutive legislation (*Family Law Act 1975* (Cth)), but also by the Australian Constitution (*MIMIA v B*, 377 [6]).

This chapter takes a critical approach to jurisdiction – the way in which bodies come to be included within law and legal authority (Dorsett & McVeigh, 2012). Legal authority and action are approached as contained in jurisdictional space, the boundaries of which determine who can be included within this jurisdiction to be acted upon by judicial decision-making (Douglas, Sarat & Umphrey, 2005). Jurisdiction has an important constitutive role because it 'empower[s] and legitimate[s]' acts of judicial – and in turn state – authority (Douglas et al., 2005, p. 9; see also pp. 10–11).

The FCA's legal authority to authorise sterilisation is grounded in its 'welfare jurisdiction' and hence is legally bounded by the well-being of children and, in constitutional terms, by the child's well-being in the context of the parent–child relationship. To analyse the welfare jurisdiction, I draw on Alison Kafer's (2013) concept of the 'curative imaginary'. Kafer (2013) has argued that where 'disability is conceptualised as a terrible unending tragedy ... [a] better future ... is one that excludes disability and disabled bodies' (p. 2). As such, therapeutic interventions (including sterilisation) become understood and accepted within a 'curative imaginary': 'an understanding of disability that not only *expects* and *assumes* intervention but also cannot imagine or comprehend anything other than intervention' (p. 27; emphasis added). Eunjung Kim (2016) refers to therapeutic interventions as forms of 'curative violence', being violent in the double sense of the physical intervention and the negation of the inherent value of the disabled subject. The 'curative' encourages us to question the self-evidence of the FCA's role in sterilisation, notably the centrality of well-being.

In taking a critical approach to jurisdiction and disability, I explore how the judiciary is positioned to legitimately permit the violence of sterilisation by examining the majority judgments in the leading HCA decisions on court-authorised sterilisation. These decisions are *Marion's Case*, which established that the FCA has authority to authorise sterilisation by reason of its welfare jurisdiction, and *P v P* (1994) 181 CLR 583, which affirmed the FCA's jurisdiction despite state guardianship laws utilising stricter criteria in determining whether to authorise sterilisation.

My core argument is that the legitimacy of the judiciary's role in the lawful violence of sterilisation is attributable to a curative imaginary underpinning the majority's approach to the FCA's welfare jurisdiction. This curative imaginary is apparent in three respects. The first (as envisioned by Kafer) is that the majority in each decision determines that sterilisation is unquestionably necessary to enhance disabled girls' well-being. The two further respects which I propose move beyond what is anticipated by Kafer, and instead cast Kafer's approach to curative imaginary in the specific context of jurisdiction and legality and the relationship between disability and law. Acknowledging judicial authority to permit sterilisation both shores up limits and gaps in the scope of state authority vis-à-vis disabled girls' bodies and individualises and privatises the injustices of sterilisation. I conclude that de-legitimising the judiciary's role in sterilisation requires contesting curative assumptions about disability and law. This chapter's analysis signals the need for greater engagement with discourses of humanitarianism, care and flourishing, particularly when these discourses are mobilised by law in coercive and violent contexts against people with disability and a wider variety of marginalised populations.

Marion's Case

Marion's Case arose out of an application by 'Marion's' parents for the FCA to authorise their daughter's hysterectomy and oophorectomy.[1] At first instance, Chief Justice Nicholson stated a case for the opinion of the Full Court of the FCA on whether Marion's parents could lawfully authorise her sterilisation without a court order and if not what was the scope of the FCA's jurisdiction (*Marion's Case*, pp. 229–230). The Full Court of the FCA (*In Re Marion* (1990) 14 Fam LR 427) was split on whether court authorisation was required. The case was then appealed to the HCA.

The majority (Chief Justice Mason and Justices Dawson, Toohey and Gaudron) held that the FCA has jurisdiction to authorise parental consent to sterilisation pursuant to its welfare jurisdiction. The majority began by noting that court authorisation was necessary because decisions on sterilisation were prone to societal prejudices about disability (pp. 238–239). Moreover, there was a significant risk of a wrong decision being made by parents because of the 'complexity of the question of consent' (p. 250), the medicalisation of the decision to sterilise by reason of the 'central role' of the medical profession (p. 251), the potential for 'conflicting (though legitimate) interests of the parents and other family members' (p. 251) and the 'gravity of the consequences of wrongly authorising a sterilisation' (p. 252). The majority also premised their view that court authorisation was required on the right to personal inviolability[2] (pp. 253–254). Thus, even before identifying the specific court or jurisdiction responsible for authorising sterilisation, the majority positions the judiciary as *protector* of disabled girls' safety and personal integrity: at a fundamental level the judiciary is positioned as non-violent (Steele, 2014).

The majority then turned to identify the 'welfare jurisdiction' as empowering the FCA to decide on sterilisation (pp. 254–260). The majority likened the welfare jurisdiction to the 'parens patriae jurisdiction' (p. 256),[3] describing it as being 'founded on the *obvious necessity* that the law should place somewhere the care of individuals who cannot take care of themselves, particularly in cases where *it is clear* that some care should be thrown round them' (*Wellesley v Duke of Beaufort* (1827) 2 Russ 1 at 20, cited at 258; emphasis added). As such, the majority characterises the relationship between the FCA and disabled girls in terms of care and dependency and characterise disabled girls as inevitably in need of the court's interventions. In doing so, sterilisation (and the judiciary itself) is positioned as non-violent. The apparent self-evidence underpinning the majority's discussion hints at a curative imaginary of disabled girls (in the sense Kafer anticipated) because the majority positions intervention as absolute. Moreover, this self-evidence conceals questions about the judiciary's role in the legality of interventions in disabled girls' bodies in the absence of explicit and specific legislative powers (i.e., the second sense of 'curative imaginary' I identified in the introduction), a point I will further explore in my later discussion of Justice Brennan's dissenting opinions in *Marion's Case* and *P v P* below.

The majority then considered 'the precise function of a court in relation to authorising sterilisation', stating that it is 'within narrow confines' and is a 'step of last resort' and should ultimately be about protecting the child in order to maximise their life possibilities:

> The *objective to be secured by sterilisation is the welfare of the disabled child*. Within that context, it is apparent that sterilisation can *only be authorised* in the case of a child so disabled that other procedures or treatments are or have proved inadequate in the sense that they have failed or will not alleviate the situation so that the *child can lead a life in keeping with his or her needs and capacities.*
>
> ... if authorisation is given, it will not be on account of the convenience of sterilisation as a contraceptive measure, but because it is *necessary to enable her to lead a life in keeping with her needs and capacities.*
>
> (pp. 259–260; emphasis added)

This statement by the majority only makes sense pursuant to a curative imaginary of disability. The sterilisation procedure is necessary to unlock a life that disabled girls would otherwise be unable to access because of their disability. Yet at the same time, this future life is ultimately still constrained by that same disability ('keeping with her needs and capacities'). The 'good' life or better future for disabled girls realised through sterilisation is in fact one which denies to them many of the very life experiences such as menstruation, reproduction and parenting which are associated with 'normal' female life experience. While these life experiences are arguably culturally constructed to render 'normal females' deficient vis-à-vis males, girls with disability are viewed as hyper-risky and unruly because they are incapable of managing these experiences in a socially appropriate way. As such, it is not so much that girls are literally cured of their disability through court-authorised sterilisation, but that their disability prompts *an impulse to cure* (regardless of the outcome). It is this impulse to cure which masks both the violence and harmful outcomes of the intervention and the reinscribing of biopolitical rule over the disabled girl's body. This suggests that contesting the legitimacy of judicial authority in sterilisation requires advancing a 'different mode of relation to life' (Golder, 2015, p. 129) which does not fold back into curative understandings of the disabled 'good life'.[4]

The legitimacy of FCA authorisation was ultimately bounded by Constitutional authority. As I will explain, this is problematic because of the Court's narrow and technical approach to the scope of Constitutional authority, which largely overlooked individual rights or broader ethical, social and political considerations. The Australian Constitution constrains and distributes powers of government within a federal system consisting of Commonwealth and state/territory governments. Section 51 of the Constitution establishes the power of the Australian government to legislate in relation to specific areas (referred to as 'heads of power'). In order for the FCA as a judicial arm of the Australian government to have the authority pursuant to its welfare jurisdiction to order sterilisation, the welfare jurisdiction as contained in the *Family Law Act 1975* (Cth) must fall within a head of power under section 51. Two such powers are: 'marriage' (s 51(xxi)) and 'divorce and matrimonial causes; and in relation thereto, parental rights, and the custody and guardianship of infants' (s 51(xxii)). These heads of power enable the Commonwealth to legislate in relation to matters pertaining to parental relationship with children. Moreover, states have all used the referral power in the Australian Constitution to refer state jurisdiction over children not of a marriage to the Family Court (see, e.g., *Commonwealth Powers (Family Law) Act 1986* (NSW)). So, the HCA was concerned with whether the FCA's authorisation of sterilisation pursuant to its welfare jurisdiction fell within these heads of power. The majority was of the view that 'any limitation on the jurisdiction of the Family Court ... must be constitutional' because the *Family Law Act 1975* (Cth) 'is limited in its operation by reference to the constitutional powers under which it is enacted: "Marriage" (s 51(xxi)); "Divorce and matrimonial causes; and in relation thereto, parental rights, and the custody and guardianship of infants" (s 51(xxii))' (p. 261). Yet, the majority stated that 'the scope of the jurisdiction will nevertheless be very wide' and that '[s]o long as an order of the Family Court *is constitutional*', state legislatures cannot limit its scope (p. 261; emphasis added). Thus, the authority of the FCA to decide on sterilisation is fundamentally linked to the founding legal document of state authority – the Australian Constitution. In taking this approach to the FCA's authority over disabled girls' bodies, the HCA looks at judicial authority in a particular (narrow) way which forecloses other ways of thinking about the state (and judiciary's) relationship to disabled girls' bodies and the violence done to them through sterilisation.

This focus on constitutionality means that 'welfare' pertains specifically to the parent–child relationship as grounded in the sexual dyad of the parents, and is only legally relevant because of the technical legislative heads of power rather than because of an inherent concern for the welfare of children or, indeed, the rights of children per se. While the majority began its judgment with lofty recognition of the right to personal inviolability, there was no meaningful connection made between this general right and the actual scope of the FCA's jurisdiction. This signals the need for a more sustained examination of sterilisation in relation to constitutional law (see, however, in response to *P v P*: Ford, 1996), building on feminist critiques of constitutional law (see, e.g., Karpin & O'Connell, 2005). Australia's absence of explicit constitutional rights heightens the urgency of such an analysis, because it signals the broader reach of legitimate judicial authority and state 'irresponsibility' (Veitch, 2007) vis-à-vis disabled girls' bodies.

Turning specifically to authorisation of sterilisation in *Marion's Case*, the majority noted that:

> It is *clear enough* that a question of sterilisation of a child of a marriage arises out of the marriage relationship and that the sterilisation of a child arises from the custody or guardianship of a child. Therefore, jurisdiction to authorise sterilisation is within the reach of power of the Commonwealth …
>
> (p. 261; emphasis added)

Here the majority again rests on the seeming self-evidence of sterilisation as parental care and as part of the broader legal approach to the authority of parents to consent to their children's medical treatment. Building on the feminist family law scholarship which has criticised the privatising effect of family law (Boyd, 1999, pp. 377–382), I argue that legally bounding *judicial authority* in the parent–child relationship and the sexual dyad of the parents effectively individualises and privatises the failure of the state to provide appropriate support and resources to disabled girls and hence *cures state irresponsibility* (the third form of the curative imaginary proposed in the introduction). This particular curative aspect of the welfare jurisdiction shows an important relationship between the judiciary and the executive/legislature in relation to systemic harms and injustice experienced by disabled girls. I return to this point further below in my discussion of *MIMIA v B*. Before this, however, I consider the High Court's decision in *P v P*.

P v P

The majority judgment in *Marion's Case* was affirmed in the subsequent HCA decision of *P v P*. This decision had its origins in 'Lessli's' mother's application to the FCA for authorisation of her consent to Lessli's hysterectomy.[5] The matter was referred to the HCA as a case stated on the questions of the relationship between the FCA's jurisdiction and state-based guardianship legislation, notably whether the FCA's welfare jurisdiction extended to authorising sterilisation of a person unable to consent when this would otherwise be prohibited pursuant to state law. This was on the basis that Part 5 of the *Guardianship Act 1987* (NSW) already provided a scheme for special medical treatment (including sterilisation) and imposed 'particularly stringent restrictions' as compared with the FCA's jurisdiction (p. 596). Section 35 of the *Guardianship Act* prohibited medical treatment done otherwise than pursuant to Part 5.

The majority in *P v P* (Chief Justice Mason, and Justices Deane, Toohey and Gaudron) approached their decision by reference to a constitutional law analysis of the welfare jurisdiction – specifically whether the state guardianship laws override Commonwealth welfare jurisdiction. They were of the view that authorising 'medical treatment of an incapable child of a marriage' is 'directly related to the protection and welfare of the particular child and which arises out of, and is itself an aspect of, the relevant marriage relationship' (p. 600). As such the provisions of the *Family Law Act 1975* (Cth) conferring jurisdiction to give or withhold such authorisation 'are a law with respect to marriage within s 51(xxi) of the *Constitution*' and are 'directly concerned with parental rights and the custody and guardianship of infants in relation to divorce or matrimonial causes and are accordingly within the grant of legislative power contained in s 51(xxii)' (pp. 600–601). There is a circularity to this reasoning – even though the sterilisation is a non-therapeutic procedure, simply because the child's parents desire the procedure to be done the sterilisation is assumed to be related to the child's protection and welfare, and on this basis arises from the marriage relationship. Thus, in a similar vein to the majority in *Marion's Case*, the majority simply assumes that sterilisation is related to parenting of disabled girls (in viewing it as a medical procedure) and, additionally, that the matter need only be considered by reference to narrow textual constitutional technicalities rather than broader ethical and social considerations: so long as sterilisation fits within a head of power, its ethical, social or political legitimacy per se is largely irrelevant.

The majority were of the view that the *Guardianship Act's* section 35 prohibition was not an 'absolute prohibition' as part of the ordinary criminal law, but was prohibited by reason of the operation of the statutory scheme. Therefore, in itself the guardianship legislation did not preclude the FCA's jurisdiction to permit sterilisation that was otherwise prohibited by the guardianship legislation (p. 603), and orders made in the exercise of the federal jurisdiction would prevail over the state legislative prohibition. They noted that the *Family Law Act 1975* (Cth) made exception for children under state welfare laws, but otherwise there was no legislative intent that the FCA's welfare jurisdiction should be subject to every prohibition and constraint in state laws (p. 606). By dealing with the relationship between the welfare jurisdiction and the state guardianship legislation by reference to constitutional legal technicalities, the majority overlooked greater recognition of rights under guardianship legislation (particularly focused on protecting people with disability from violence and exploitation)[6] and, in turn, the likely very different and potentially better *material* outcome for disabled girls under guardianship schemes (Ford, 1996). Broader political and ethical issues of disability rights were rendered redundant to the narrow question of state authority as constitutional legality.

Read together, majority judgments in *Marion's Case* and *P v P* position the state, through the judiciary, as legitimately permitting the violence of sterilisation by resting on a curative imaginary which assumes that authorising sterilisation could be necessary to enhance the girls' well-being and futures, assumes that limits and gaps in the scope of state authority vis-à-vis disabled girls bodies should be filled by a general judicial power grounded on the assumed 'welfare' of intervention in their bodies, and individualises and privatises the injustices of sterilisation to the responsibility of parents. Constitutional law serves a key role in sustaining this curative imaginary, which is curative in relation to disability *and* at the nexus of disability and law. In order to further explore this more expansive reading of the curative imaginary, I turn to Justice Brennan's dissents in *Marion's Case* and *P v P*.

The instability of judicial authority

To this day, the majority judgments in *Marion's Case* and *P v P* provide the legal basis for the FCA's jurisdiction to authorise parental consent to sterilisation. However, as I now propose, this judicial authority is inherently unstable and should be the site for contesting the violence done to disabled girls through sterilisation. In this part I draw on Justice Brennan's dissenting judgments in *Marion's Case* and *P v P*, and briefly touch upon *MIMIA v B*, in order to illuminate the problematic assumptions about sterilisation as 'curative' of disabled girls, but also further highlight the relationships between the 'curative' of disability, incomplete legal authority and state irresponsibility.

In *Marion's Case* and *P v P*, Justice Brennan opposed the FCA having jurisdiction over sterilisation other than for the purpose of 'therapeutic medical treatment' (*Marion's Case*, p. 274). Justice Brennan argued in *Marion's Case* that:

> the rule must give priority to the right to physical integrity and the human dignity it protects, even though such a rule imposes burdens on parents, guardians and those having the care of the intellectually disabled child who are entitled to the active support of the State which must bear the ultimate burden.
>
> (p. 277)

Interestingly, like the majority in *Marion's Case*, he began his reasons by reference to rights, but, as I will argue, unlike the majority, he saw these rights as an important *constraint* on the scope of judicial authority. In *P v P*, Justice Brennan stated:

> Courts are instruments of State power. Unless driven by legal impera-
> tives, I would deny to any instrument of the State the power to authorise
> the invasion of the physical integrity of any person except to save that
> person's life or to save her from serious bodily harm. In particular, I
> would deny to any officer of the State the power to say: 'This invasion is
> not to save you from death or bodily harm but it is for your own welfare
> as I, the agent of the State, see it.' ... Courts and judges, in the absence of
> governing legal principle or of guidelines more specific than 'welfare' to
> control the exercise of such a daunting power, can rely only on their
> idiosyncratic perceptions of the circumstances ... When the scope of the
> welfare jurisdiction is undefined by the *Family Law Act*, I am unable to
> construe the bare term 'welfare' in such a way as to arm a judge with
> power to make an order authorising a serious and irreversible invasion of
> personal integrity.
>
> (p. 612)

In further support of this point, Justice Brennan stated that the rationale that the welfare jurisdiction should be extended to authorise sterilisation because it was in the best interests of the child 'runs counter to the fundamental common law principle of personal inviolability' which, he argued, Part 5 of the *Guardianship Act* protected (pp. 612–613). In so doing, Justice Brennan makes apparent the contradiction inherent in judicial authority being grounded in 'welfare' when the exercise of this judicial authority enables interventions that violate fundamental rights of disabled girls. In so doing, he challenges the impulse of the curative imaginary that disabled girls' welfare *necessitates* intervention.

Justice Brennan also suggested in *Marion's Case* that resort to the welfare jurisdiction reflected the limits of state authority over disabled girls, and was an attempt by the court not merely to legitimise interventions in girls' bodies but to fill gaps in law's authority. He stated:

> The hypothesis that a court is empowered to authorise the non-therapeutic
> sterilisation of intellectually disabled children is asserted in order to
> satisfy what the *court perceives to be a lacuna in the powers* which ought
> to be available to satisfy the exigencies of the situation of some disabled
> children. But the court is an instrument of State power, and the powers of
> the State to authorise interference with the personal integrity of any of its
> subjects otherwise than for therapeutic purposes is *not self-evident*.
>
> (pp. 283–284; emphasis added)

Similarly, in *P v P*, Justice Brennan was critical of the assumption that gaps in legal authority of disabled girls' bodies must be filled by granting broad judicial authority to the FCA. He explained:

> In construing 'welfare' in Pt VII in order to ascertain whether it imports a power in a judge of the Family Court to make a sterilisation order, it is not appropriate, in my respectful opinion, to begin with the proposition that, since parents and guardians cannot consent to the procedure, there *must be* power in a court to authorise the non-therapeutic sterilisation of a child. It is fallacious to start with an assumption that, in default of any other competent repository, the *power must be reposed in a court*. In principle, it is erroneous to assume that a power is reposed in a court *merely because it is thought desirable or convenient* that the power be available … Courts have the function of declaring the law, including the law which confers and governs their jurisdiction, but *they cannot enhance their powers* in order to give effect to a view that the enhancement is needed.
>
> (p. 617; emphasis added)

Justice Brennan went on to note that the principle that courts cannot assume new powers which are not part of their inherent or traditional jurisdiction or conferred by legislation is 'at the heart of the political and constitutional theory of the separation of powers and thus an important guarantee of a free society' (p. 617) and that if courts were to assume such powers 'the assumed powers would be despotic, uncontrolled by legislative prescription or other law' (p. 618). His Honour noted this was particularly the case in the context of the welfare jurisdiction and sterilisation, which could enable courts to simply override a fundamental human right:

> If the general law protects the physical integrity of incompetent children and prohibits their parents or guardians from subjecting them to non-therapeutic sterilisation, it is indeed a curious thing that a court should so interpret 'welfare' as to assert a power to authorise their subjection to that procedure, declaring the power to be a 'procedural safeguard' of the child's welfare.
>
> (p. 618)

Justice Brennan's discussion of the welfare jurisdiction as shoring up gaps in legal authority over disabled girls speaks directly to the ways that the majority judgments in *Marion's Case* and *P v P* harness a curative imaginary at the nexus of disability and law. Indeed, his discussion calls out the ways that this curative imaginary of disability *and* law works to position the state, through the judiciary, as legitimately permitting the violence of sterilisation by assuming that limits and gaps in the scope of state authority vis-à-vis disabled girls bodies *should* necessarily be filled by a general judicial power.

In *P v P* Justice Brennan also criticised the majority in *Marion's Case* on the issue of sterilisation clearly arising out of the marriage relationship. He noted that the:

> occasion for authorising the sterilisation of a child arises simply because the child is incompetent and *nobody else has power to authorise the sterilisation*. That 'occasion' does not arise out of a marriage relationship or because a child is a child of a marriage.
> (p. 626; emphasis added; see similarly Dawson J in *P v P* 628–631)

Here Justice Brennan problematises the specific constitutional bounding of the welfare jurisdiction by reference to the parent–child relationship (which in turn is grounded in the sexual dyad between the parents) as a façade, because ultimately what is being addressed is an absence of authority that anyone (parent or otherwise) has over the disabled girls' body vis-à-vis sterilisation. My analysis signals a recurring instability and uncertainty of law in relation to disabled girls' bodies. I suggest that we might view the two cases stated (both initiated by the state) on the specific question of the FCA's jurisdiction in relation to sterilisation as attempts to use the High Court to shore up the 'incompleteness' of state and legal authority over disabled girls' bodies. Yet, through the majority decisions in each of these decisions (and their enduring precedential value), the disabled girls' body has been (tenuously) refolded into jurisdiction and state authority. This refolding is perhaps taken as self-evident because the abjected visceral excess typically associated with disabled girls' bodies in sterilisation decisions (e.g., leaking menstrual blood, sexual promiscuity, erratic behaviour; on the corporeal excesses of disabled bodies, see Shildrick, 2009) intersects with their abstract legal excess to jurisdiction in order to readily rationalise intervention as necessary to bring the disabled girls' body back into legal and physical authority.

It is important to pause to consider the implications on legal authority of sterilisation's gendered nature. As per my earlier observations, it is disabled girls' bodies that are seen as more dangerous in their inability to be contained and managed and hence it is disabled girls (and their sexuality) who present a much greater threat to legal order than disabled boys. The disabled girls' body suggests the fragility of legal authority by pushing the state to the point of seeking HCA guidance on the jurisdictional status of their bodies, and hence indicates new openings for political and theoretical engagement with law's complicity in sterilisation.

Brennan J's dissenting comments are not only important for illuminating the problematic reliance on the welfare jurisdiction to violate girls' rights, but for showing the politically productive possibilities of disability in illuminating the limits of state's lawful authority over marginal bodies. 'Welfare' can be critiqued as functioning in its emptiness to both shore up law's gaps of authority to retrieve this excess to lawful authority (Shildrick, 2009) and reclaim its 'completeness' – that no one is above or beyond the law (as per Golder & Fitzpatrick, 2009; see Carter, 2016). Yet, as per Shildrick (2009), disability might have a disruptive potential in relation to state authorisation of violence through court-mandated treatment; scholars and activists can engage with the question of whether disability can threaten law's illimitability.

This brings us to the third form of curative imaginary: that judicial authorisation of sterilisation 'cures' the injustice of sterilisation. Justice Brennan noted in both *Marion's Case* and *P v P* that court authorisation would leave children with no redress against the judge or medical practitioners for their sterilisation (*Marion's Case*, pp. 283–284; *P v P*, pp. 612–613). This suggests that we need to question how the role of the court in authorising sterilisation alters our ability to read this as an injustice, and what the implications might be for redress. Further than issues of individual injustice, legally bounding *judicial authority* in the parent–child relationship effectively individualises and privatises the failure of the state to provide appropriate support and resources to disabled girls and hence *cures systemic state irresponsibility*.

This point of systemic (as opposed to individual) irresponsibility is further supported by the more recent decision of *MIMIA v B. MIMIA v B* concerned orders sought pursuant to the welfare jurisdiction by parents of children in immigration detention to have their children released from 'indefinite' immigration detention on the basis that 'their continued detention was harmful to their welfare' (p. 365). It was unanimously held by the HCA that the orders sought were not within the jurisdiction of the FCA. Chief Justice Gleeson and Justice Murray held that the FCA has no jurisdiction to make orders directing the release of children or in relation to their welfare in immigration detention (p. 375 [1]) because the welfare jurisdiction is generally concerned with 'the relationship between parents and children and parents' duties in respect of their children' (p. 390 [52]; see similarly Justices Gummow, Hayne, Callinan & Heydon, pp. 406–407 [110]; Justice Callinan [215] 439). In this decision in *MIMIA v B*, the HCA not only demonstrated that issues pertaining to a child's well-being, safety and vulnerability in public and state contexts is not a welfare issue, but both place principal responsibility on parents for children's welfare and carve out a space for state irresponsibility in relation to systemic policies that are harmful or unjust to children. In this respect, the role of the judiciary in court-authorised sterilisation both frames parents (rather than the courts and the state) as principally responsible for the act of violence (courts merely authorise parents to do the act of consent) and masks systemic policy failures that position sterilisation as the solution to care and well-being issues. Therefore, the curative imaginary at work in court-authorised sterilisation simultaneously necessitates the intervention in disabled girls' bodies and negates the violence and multiple individual and systemic injustices of this intervention and access to specific legal avenues of redress (on the legal impossibility of bearing witness to and redressing institutional violence, see Chapter 6, this volume).

Conclusion

This chapter sought to examine how the HCA has reconciled the violence of sterilisation with the exercise of judicial authority grounded on child welfare. This has occurred through framing sterilisation as an issue of well-being, as an act of parental care and as a technical matter of constitutionality of judicial power. This analysis showed that in 'curing' disability, the FCA is also 'curing' law of the limits that disability presents to legal authority and 'curing' the state of the systemic irresponsibilities associated with sterilisation. Conjuring the better future and good life of disabled girls has complex legal and political implications for state authority more broadly.

Making apparent the tenuous nature of judicial authority might open a larger discussion around court-mandated interventions, disability and state authority which, rather than sitting at the margins of political thought as a 'disability' issue, cuts at the core of broader issues of illegitimacy, irresponsibility and injustice relevant to diverse marginalised groups. In particular, the analysis signals the need for close attention to the links of jurisdiction and judicial authority with the Constitution as the founding document of lawfulness of state authority. This is even more urgent in a context where there is no comprehensive constitutional protection of rights. There is a need to bring into relief the relationship between the disabled girls' body and the Constitution, and to trouble concepts of care in relation to disability, not only vis-à-vis the effects of interventions but how these order relations between marginalised individuals and the state.

In reflecting on the curative imaginary at work in the legality of the violence of sterilisation, we should look to longer continuities in the legal imagining. It is 90 years since the infamous US Supreme Court decision of *Buck v Bell* (1927) 274 U.S. 200. *Buck v Bell* is typically cited as the reference point for a period when sterilisation was done for the *wrong* reasons – for eugenics, or as Justice Deane states, 'public welfare' reasons (see, e.g., Justice Brennan, p. 275, and Justice Deane, p. 300 of *Marion's Case*). Nevertheless, to this day we can see the law drawing on normative assumptions about the (different) good life of people with disability *and* positioning the court as a non-violent arbiter on how sterilisation can achieve this life. It is vital that we make apparent and trouble these (largely unacknowledged) continuities in the role of the judiciary in the welfare and well-being of women and girls with disability.

Shifting to more recent history, while *Marion's Case* and *P v P* were decided over 20 years ago, their legacy remains ever present in legal and political discussion of sterilisation. In 2013, an Australian Senate Inquiry examined the legal framework of sterilisation pursuant to the FCA's welfare jurisdiction. The report acknowledged 'concerns around the operation and expertise of the Family Court in child sterilisation cases' and stated that '[t]he committee has seriously considered the question of whether it is appropriate for the Family

Court to continue hearing child sterilisation cases.' Yet, ultimately the report stated that 'the committee concludes that it would not be appropriate for the jurisdiction to be removed' (Senate Community Affairs References Committee 2013 p. 67 [3.50]). This was on the basis that the FCA, as a Commonwealth court, 'provides consistency for all Australian children regardless of where they live' (p. 68 [3.50]) and 'were the Family Court's jurisdiction to be removed, protections of the child will depend on where the child lives', which was of particular concern in those jurisdictions where there is no alternative legislative scheme of sterilisation (p. 68 [3.51]). The Senate Report had not moved very far from the protective judiciary envisioned by the majority in *Marion's Case*. Ultimately, the Senate Report was largely silent on questions of violence, state authority and jurisdiction. It is a challenge to us as scholars and advocates to respond to these silences.

Acknowledgements

Thank you to Nicole Wesson for her research assistance and to Felicity Bell, Isabel Karpin, Kate Seear and Claire Spivakovsky for their feedback on earlier drafts.

Notes

1 For an overview of the facts related to the sterilisation see *In re Marion (No 2)* (1992) 17 Fam LR 336.
2 The right to personal inviolability or bodily integrity privileges an individuals' autonomy over his or her body, including control over physical contact with or interventions in their body (see *Marion's Case*, pp. 233–234).
3 For an overview of the *parens patriae* jurisdiction, see Chapter 10, this volume.
4 Certainly this point has some resonance in the context of the use of the welfare jurisdiction to regulate trans children's access to hormone treatment (Bell, 2015); some of these children, as well as trans advocates and scholars, have resisted the Family Court's role in authorising treatment (although the treatment is desired, cf sterilisation which is non-desired treatment (for a critical contrasting of law's role in sterilisation and hormone treatment, see Pyne, 2017)).
5 For an overview of the facts, see *P v P* (1995) 126 FLR 245.
6 For a historical overview of guardianship legislation, see John Chesterman's chapter in this collection.

References

Bell, F. (2015). Children with gender dysphoria and the jurisdiction of the Family Court. *University of New South Wales Law Journal* 38(2), 426–454.

Boyd, S. (1999). Family, law and sexuality: Feminist engagements. *Social & Legal Studies* 8(3), 369–390.

Carter, D. (2016). HIV transmission, public health detention and the recalcitrant subject of discipline: Kuoth, Lam v R and the co-constitution of public health and criminal law. *Griffith Law Review* 25(2), 172–196.

Dorsett, S., & McVeigh, S. (2012). *Jurisdiction*. London: Routledge-Cavendish.

Douglas, L., Sarat, A., & Umphrey, M. M. (2005). At the limits of law: An introduction. In L. Douglas, A. Sarat & M. M. Umphrey (Eds.), *The limits of law* (pp. 1–20). Stanford: Stanford University Press.

Ford, J. (1996). The sterilisation of young women with an intellectual disability: A comparison between the Family Court of Australia and the Guardianship Board of New South Wales. *Australian Journal of Family Law* 10(3), 236–262.

Frohmader, C. (2013). *Dehumanised: The forced sterilisation of women and girls with disabilities in Australia*. Rosny Park: Women With Disabilities Australia.

Golder, B. (2015). *Foucault and the politics of rights*. Stanford: Stanford University Press.

Golder, B., & Fitzpatrick, P. (2009). *Foucault's law*. Abingdon & New York: Routledge.

Kafer, A. (2013). *Feminist, queer, crip*. Bloomington and Indianapolis: Indiana University Press.

Karpin, I.A., & O'Connell, K. (2005). Speaking into a silence: Embedded constitutionalism, the Australian Constitution, and the rights of women. In B. Baines & R. Rubio-Marin (Eds.), *The gender of constitutional jurisprudence* (pp. 22–47). Cambridge: Cambridge University Press.

Kim, E. (2016). *Curative violence: Rehabilitating disability, gender, and sexuality in modern Korea*. Durham and London: Duke University Press.

Pyne, J. (2017). Arresting Ashley X: Trans youth, puberty blockers and the question of whether time is on your side. *Somatechnics* 7(1), 95–123.

Senate Community Affairs References Committee (2013). *Involuntary or coerced sterilisation of people with disabilities in Australia*. Canberra: Parliament of Australia.

Shildrick, M. (2009). *Dangerous discourses of disability, subjectivity and sexuality*. Hampshire: Palgrave Macmillan.

Steele, L. (2014). Disability, abnormality and criminal law: Sterilisation as lawful and good violence. *Griffith Law Review* 23(3), 467–497.

Steele, L. (2016). Court-authorised sterilisation and human rights: Inequality, discrimination and violence against women and girls with disability? *UNSW Law Journal* 39(3), 1002–1037.

Veitch, S. (2007). *Law and irresponsibility: On the legitimation of human suffering*. Abingdon and New York: Routledge-Cavendish.

Legislation

Commonwealth Powers (Family Law) Act 1986 (NSW)
Family Law Act 1975 (Cth)
Guardianship Act 1987 (NSW)

Cases

Buck v Bell (1927) 274 U.S. 200
In Re Marion (1990) 14 Fam LR 427
Minister for Immigration, Migration and Indigenous Affairs v B (2004) 219 CLR 365 (*MIMIA v B*)
Secretary, Department of Health and Community Services v JWB (1992) 175 CLR 218 (*Marion's Case*)
Wellesley v Duke of Beaufort (1827) 2 Russ (UK)

Chapter 10

Mandated treatment for seriously ill minors

Ian Freckelton

The ethics, legality and utility of coercing patients into treatment they do not want or whose need they contest are sources of potential conflict that can involve clinicians, hospitals, the courts, parents and children. They raise profound dilemmas for law, medicine and ethics. Therapeutic jurisprudence has taught us that the use of force to make people submit to treatment and to live their lives in a particular way is often counter-productive and counter-therapeutic (Tyler, 1996; Winick, 1997). It can result in patients resisting treatment, experiencing distress, and passivity and non-involvement in treatment decision-making (see Kallert, Mezzich & Monahan, 2011). It can also contaminate the relationship between the provider and recipient of health services and preclude, or at least adversely affect, the creation or maintenance of therapeutic rapport.

When a seriously ill child is the recipient of health services and the child and/or their parents are resistant to such services, there are particularly complex issues for clinicians, child protection authorities and the courts. Traditionally, the final and binding decisions about such matters are made by superior courts 'in the child's best interests', and for the most part Supreme Court and Family Court judges have made orders authorising – although technically not mandating – treatment such as chemotherapy, radiotherapy, blood transfusions and even surgical procedures (Freckelton & McGregor, 2016; Freckelton & McGregor, 2017). However, the distinction between such authorisations and coercion in respect of treatment is subtle.

A new spotlight was shone on the issue by three high-visibility judgments by the Western Australian Family Court during 2016 in relation to six-year-old Oshin Kiszko (see further Freckelton, 2016). The facts underlying the judgments called for an in-depth analysis of what constitute a child's best interests when their parents are antagonistic toward mandated treatment on the basis of the adverse effect that such treatment may have upon the child's wellbeing and when such treatment may have a deleterious effect upon the child's quality of life. Oshin's circumstances required the court to wrestle with the question of when it is appropriate to exercise the coercive powers of a court if this would occasion antagonism and distress for the child's parents, which then would affect the emotional wellbeing of a vulnerable, possibly dying child. The case also raised the issue of the lengths to which it is appropriate for courts – in the exercise of their best interest powers – to mandate treatment when the prospects of success in such treatment are only moderate and when its side effects may be significant.

This chapter contextualises the decision-making in the Kiszko judgments within the generally paternalistic approach of the law in relation to the exercise of coercive powers to attempt to save a minor's life by imposing treatment which they, and/or their parents, are purporting to decline. It argues that the starting point of decision-making should be a collaborative avoidance of the deployment of force, but if opposition to potentially life-saving treatment is not in a child's best interest, robust and prompt action and curial decision-making should take place so as to maximise the prospects of as good an outcome as is feasible.

The orthodox legal position

In multiple cases brought before Australian Supreme Courts prior to the Kiszko litigation, orders had been made as part of their *parens patriae* jurisdiction to safeguard the interests of the vulnerable (see, e.g., *Secretary, Department of Health and Community Services*, 1992), including in respect of potentially life-saving treatment (see, e.g., *Minister for Health v AS*, 2004; *Children, Youth & Family Services Inc v YJL*, 2010; *X v Sydney Children's Hospital Network*, 2013). On several occasions treatment resistance arose from the parents and children being Jehovah's Witnesses and therefore opposed to the administration of others' blood products. On other occasions issues have arisen internationally by reason of parents' antagonism toward orthodox medicine or a desire for alternative forms of treatment (see, in the United Kingdom, *Re King (A Child)* (2014); *Great Ormond Street Hospital for Children NHS Foundation Trust v Yates*, 2017; in New Zealand, Liam Williams-Holloway, who was taken to Mexico contrary to court orders (Carter et al., 2002); in Australia, Laura Boomsma, who was taken from Queensland to England to receive high doses of intravenous vitamin C with dendritic cell therapy, a process designed to stimulate white blood cells to destroy cancerous cells – see Adams, 2002). Australian courts have held that the entitlement to countermand the wishes of a child patient or of their parents should be exercised sparingly, but generally preservation of a child's life, even at the cost of breaching religious beliefs or infringing on parents' autonomy as to selection of treatment, has been held to be in the child's best interests.

Prior to the Kiszko decisions, the courts had acknowledged that the reasons for opposition to treatment were relevant to the exercise of the courts' powers (see, e.g., *X v Sydney Children's Hospital Network*, 2013), accepted that respect should be accorded to the dignity of religious and other beliefs (see, e.g., *Hospital v T*, 2015), and agreed that 'best interests' include more than a child's physical wellbeing (see, e.g., *Children, Youth & Family Services Inc v YJL*, 2010), but 'sanctity of life' had weighed heavily in decision-making (see, e.g., *Children, Youth & Family Services Inc v YJL*, 2010; *Hospital v T*, 2015; *X v Sydney Children's Hospital Network*, 2013).

An influential English decision (*The NHS Trust v A (A Child)*, 2008) dealt with whether complex operative procedures should be undertaken on a child with a craniofacial sarcoma. Justice Mostyn held that the concept of 'best interests' needs to be interpreted broadly so as to comprehend medical, emotional, sensory (pleasure, pain and suffering) and instinctive (the human instinct to survive) considerations, but giving considerable weight to the 'very strong presumption' to prolong life. He observed that a variety of considerations can affect the views of parents and their children in such situations. He went further in terms of the balance between the expression of wishes by parents and children and the courts' responsibility, concluding that:

> Their own wishes, however understandable in human terms, are wholly irrelevant to consideration of the objective best interests of the child save to the extent in any given case that they may illuminate the quality and value to the child of the child/parent relationship.
>
> (at [14])

This led Justice Mostyn to arrive emphatically at the conclusion that the craniofacial surgery on the child should proceed:

> I give full weight to the wishes of J as well as those of his parents. It is a strong thing for me, a stranger, to disagree with and override the wishes of J and his parents. But I have absolutely no doubt that J must be given the chance, a very good chance, of a long and fulfilling life rather than suffering, quite soon, a ghastly, agonising, death.
>
> (at [15])

The Oshin Kiszko litigation

In a sequence of three judgments in March, May and September 2016 (*Kiszko 1, Kiszko 2* and *Kiszko 3*), Chief Justice Thackray and Justice O'Brien of the Family Court of Western Australia dealt with the circumstances of a young child, Oshin Kiszko (Oshin), who was diagnosed with a medulloblastoma, a rare brain tumour, which was removed in December 2015. However, there was the potential for fatal recurrence of the tumour and the side effects of the potentially prophylactic treatment deeply troubled his parents. This led to the convening of the hospital ethics committee, at which the medical practitioners and the parents were given an opportunity to explain their respective positions in respect of whether Oshin should receive further treatment for his condition and, if so, what that further treatment should be.

The doctors' view was that a combination of chemotherapy and radio-therapy was clinically advisable. However, Oshin's mother explained that because of her own situation of having experienced chronic back pain and her consequent inability to support Oshin's weight, which was important to the care he would need away from the hospital, she opposed the medical practi-tioners' proposal. Oshin's mother also expressed concerns arising from her own life experience of close family members who had died of cancer. She held qualifications in natural therapies and stated that she wanted to try herbal remedies for a time. By contrast, the clinicians contended that chemotherapy and radiotherapy needed to be administered urgently to minimise the chance of Oshin's cancer cells proliferating. The parents were also interested in pur-suing treatment in the United States in the form of medicinal cannabis, the efficacy of which in such a context was unproven.

Thackray CJ concluded that, from an ethical perspective, decisions needed to be made in Oshin's best interest:

> To this extent, parental autonomy may be limited. The difficulty is that a child's best interest is often not an absolute, but an assessment that will be heavily influenced by the beliefs and experience of any individual or body considering the issue. Another ethical principle is to consider such matters in terms of the burdens and benefits of any proposed line of treatment. Again, both burdens and benefits are perceptions that an adult must consider on behalf of a child.
>
> (*Kiszko 1*, at [30])

The ethics committee strongly encouraged the doctors and the family to continue an open dialogue to work toward common ground, and its members expressed the aspiration that the prescribed medical therapies could be given in conjunction with natural remedies in which Oshin's mother had faith. However, by March 2016 the family was withholding consent for 'standard therapy' and actively rejecting conventional treatments, significantly reducing the prospects for Oshin's recovery from the perspective of his doctors. Oshin's mother said that the family felt pressured by a 'dismal diagnosis' and had formed the view that the proposed treatment would not be in Oshin's best interests.

The committee's view about Oshin's mother's proposal was that it was not a rational approach and was not supported by the available scientific evidence: 'While consenting adults are free to choose such paths for themselves, it is ethically indefensible to impose such irrational beliefs on the lives of others and there are legal avenues that serve to protect children under these circum-stances' (*Kiszko 1*, at [38]). Chief Justice Thackray emphasised that an ethics committee is 'but one part of a decision-making process and it is not deter-minative of the process' (*Kiszko 1*, at [34]), but took its views into account. He noted that a treatment decision had become 'time critical' because Oshin's disease had progressed and the tumour was on the cusp of a 'massive and irreversible progression, suggesting that it is critical that the boy commences treatment with curative intent urgently' *(Kiszko 1*, at [45]). He applied prior judgments of Australian courts in relation to the provision of blood products to Jehovah's Witness children who conscientiously objected, noting that the evidence before him made it clear, beyond all doubt, that:

> Oshin will die within a few months if measures are not taken to prevent his death. The evidence indicates that there is about a 30 per cent prospect of survival after five years if he undertakes the chemotherapy that could commence tomorrow.
>
>   The evidence further indicates that there is a probability in the range of 50 per cent that if he has both chemotherapy and radiotherapy, he will be alive in five years' time. Those statistics, given by experts of considerable experience and expertise, indicate to me that there is 'a good prospect of a long-term cure'.
>
> *(Kiszko 1*, at [78]-[80])

Chief Justice Thackray took account of the wishes of Oshin's parents, accepting that they had tried to approach the matter on the basis of what was in Oshin's best interests. He acknowledged they were correct in saying that:

> of all people, they would be able to observe matters relating to their child that others would not. But, on the other hand, I also consider that there is wisdom in what was said in the deliberations of the Ethics Committee about the difficulty for parents to see beyond the immediate short to medium term negative impact of the treatment upon the quality of life of the child against the prospect that there is a cure possibly available.
>
> *(Kiszko* 1, at [81])

However, he concluded that the prospect of a long-term cure was the consideration that needed to weigh most heavily in his analysis, and ordered Oshin's treatment to commence the next week *(Kiszko 1*, at [82]). He commented that another matter which should be given weight was that the uncontested medical evidence showed the great majority of other parents faced with a similar decision would opt for the intervention the hospital proposed *(Kiszko 1*, at [83]).

   Chief Justice Thackray's March decision enabled Oshin's chemotherapy to commence, and an opportunity was given for his parents to adduce further evidence before the start of radiotherapy about whether that component of the treatment should proceed. After a further hearing some seven weeks later, Chief Justice Thackray ruled on the radiotherapy question in Kiszko 2, noting that by then Oshin had submitted to two courses of chemotherapy. The results demonstrated that there had been a significant reduction in the size of cancerous nodules in Oshin's brain, but only a very minor response in the area where the disease originated. The results also revealed 'degenerate small cells' in the cerebrospinal fluid that had the potential to be cancerous.

In giving evidence during the *Kiszko 2* litigation, the head of paediatric oncology expressed the view that Oshin's level of response was such that further chemotherapy alone would not save his life, and that a high-level dose of radiotherapy in conjunction with chemotherapy was required if Oshin was to have a realistic chance of survival. He expressed the opinion that those chances had now reduced to around 30–40% if the treatment was undertaken promptly. His prognosis was difficult to gauge because the delay in the commencement of treatment (caused by Oshin's parents' opposition to treatment and the time taken to institute and resolve the legal proceedings) had placed him well outside the range of the sample groups used to make predictions. However, Chief Justice Thackray framed the doctor's view as being: 'he will be likely to die within months unless treated' (*Kiszko 2*, at [12]).

Oshin's parents continued to resist chemotherapy right up until the radiotherapy hearing, even erecting a 'Forced Chemo' sign above Oshin's hospital bed, and sometimes refusing to assist nursing staff in caring for and comforting Oshin. However, they complied with the court order. Shortly before the hearing, a forensic report from an interstate paediatric oncologist, commissioned by Oshin's parents, Professor K, became available. It recommended additional chemotherapy, but opined that the parents' opposition to radiotherapy should be respected given the risks of harm to his developing brain that it posed to Oshin. In light of Professor K's views, the parents abandoned their previous position and said that they now wished Oshin to have the further chemotherapy treatment recommended by Professor K, but not radiotherapy.

Professor K expressed the view that the results of the most recent MRI suggested that the prospect that Oshin would be a long-term survivor, even if he had chemotherapy and radiotherapy, was less than 40–50%. It was also his view that the chances of negative effects from radiation therapy, including depression of intellect, were high (*Kiszko 2*, at [39]).

Chief Justice Thackray observed that the dilemma in striking the right balance in making decisions about the treatment of life-threatening illnesses is even more acute and agonising when the life is that of a child: 'that dilemma, and the deeply held conviction of Oshin's parents that the quality of life should be prioritized over its duration, is at the heart of this case' (*Kiszko 2*, at [48]). He noted that the real difference between the medical practitioners was that Professor K placed greater emphasis on the long-term quality of life of Oshin, whereas the hospital doctors placed greater emphasis on the maintenance of life itself. The other important apparent difference of opinion was that Professor K held out some hope that a continuation of the chemotherapy might, in itself, lead to a cure for Oshin. By contrast, the hospital had virtually abandoned hope that chemotherapy would ensure Oshin's survival.

Chief Justice Thackray stated that he agreed with the decision of Justice Tompkins in the New Zealand decision of *Re Norma* (1992):

> welfare is not to be regarded in only a physical or medical context, although undoubtedly those will be important. A child's welfare is also bound up with his or her family. If a course of action is likely to cause serious distress and disruption within a family, that too is a factor that must bear on the welfare of the child and therefore weigh with the Court.
>
> (at 451)

He affirmed the proposition that the court's power to countermand the wishes of a child's parents is to be exercised sparingly and with great caution. He noted that 'best interests' relate to values, not to facts (see *CDJ v VAJ*, 1998, at 219). This led him to observe that his decision should not be made in a vacuum but need to be made in the context of Oshin's specific circumstances:

> being a unique and important individual, but also in the context of him being a member of his own family and a member of the wider society. It is to be made also in light of the fact that ... each of Oshin's parents is invested with parental responsibility for him, which is defined as meaning 'all the duties, powers, responsibilities and authority which, by law, parents have in relation to children'. The state should not interfere in the performance of their parental obligations unless there is 'some clear justification' for doing so.
>
> (*Kiszko 2*, at [63])

This resulted in Chief Justice Thackray identifying 'two social, moral or ethical questions': the first, whether greater emphasis should be placed on life itself or on the quality of the life; and the second, whether the first question should be answered by the court as the representative of the state or by the parents, who in every other respect are permitted to make decisions on behalf of their child who is too young to make decisions for himself (*Kiszko 2*, at [65]).

Chief Justice Thackray was influenced by the fact that he was referred to no other case in which a medical intervention had been imposed in spite of a reputable independent expert opining that the views of the parents opposing the intervention were supportable based on the relative benefits and burdens of the proposed treatment. He concluded that:

> In the absence of a consensus of qualified medical opinion, there is, in my view, no role for the state in directing the parents to act in accordance with one entirely valid opinion in preference to another. My view is reinforced by the fact that at least in Professor K's clinical experience,

although it is not the experience of the doctors at PMH, a substantial minority of parents would follow the course adopted by Oshin's parents.

(Kiszko 2, at [68])

In arriving at his decision, he stated that he had also taken into account the conduct of Oshin's parents, and their passionate and highly public objection to Oshin undergoing radiotherapy:

Their behaviour gives cause for concern about their ability to control their emotions around this topic in the presence of Oshin. If Oshin were to have 'forced' radiotherapy, I fear he would again be exposed to his parents' hostility and bitterness, potentially causing him even more psychological trauma. The impact on the parents of such forced treatment is therefore itself relevant in the determination of Oshin's best interests in circumstances where his treatment regime and after-treatment care will require the intimate involvement and support of the family.

(Kiszko 2, at [71])

A further factor which he took into account was that the independent child lawyer submitted that the orders that the court should make ought to be in accordance with the views of Professor K.

Chief Justice Thackray accepted the agreement between Oshin's parents and the clinicians that Oshin should have the recommended further chemotherapy. He adjourned the hospital's application for orders in respect of radiotherapy (rather than rejecting it) and discharged the interim orders. However, this proved to be the end of neither the parents' opposition to Oshin's treatment nor the clinicians' wishes to treat Oshin with further chemotherapy and radiotherapy. Oshin's mother reported to the media that her son had developed ulcers in his stomach, and could barely eat or use the toilet. She said he lashed out at his family to try to avoid treatment. Her wish was to:

offer Oshin peace, love and some fun times while we still can … I have watched and learned what these children and their families go through and it is nothing short of toxic hell … The children are not really alive, they are completely drugged and exhausted and on the verge of death.

(MacLaughlin, 2016)

On 19 August 2016, in light of the new impasse, clinicians applied to Justice O'Brien, also of the Western Australian Family Court, for permission to administer higher-dose chemotherapy and renewed their application for radiotherapy. Oshin's parents responded by arguing that Oshin should be viewed as terminally ill and simply given palliative care. They were implacably opposed to the further pursuit of curative treatment and urged that the quality of his life should be prioritised over the duration of his life:

> They do not want him to spend the time he has left enduring curative treatment processes which have very low prospects of success. Even if the curative treatment processes were to be successful, they regard the long-term side effects of radiation therapy in particular as being too high a price to pay for longevity. They hold deeply to the belief that Oshin has a right to die with dignity and in peace.
>
> (Kiszko 3, at [65]–[66])

The expert evidence from the hospital conceded that the prospects of cure for Oshin with consolidation chemotherapy had become less than 10%, but argued that a combination of the therapies constituted his best prospect of cure. Meanwhile, the interstate expert oncologist called on behalf of Oshin's parents expressed the view that, whatever could now be done, because of the delays, Oshin's chances of survival had become 'remote'. (Kiszko 3, at [53])

On 1 September 2016, Justice O'Brien ruled on the third application. He commented that 'regardless of the exercise of parental responsibility per se the child's welfare and best interests are inextricably entwined with his role as a member of his family' (*Kiszko 3,* at [82]). He held that the Family Court was obliged to exercise caution in countermanding parental decisions and should do so only sparingly (*Kiszko 3*, at [84]). He took into account the 'clear deterioration in Oshin's prospects of a cure' over the previous months and the emphatic and deeply held views of his parents as to what was best for him:

> The importance to Oshin of his relationship with his parents weighs heavily in my decision. That relationship, and the support and love which only his parents can give, are of critical importance to Oshin and to his quality of life over the months to come. I am deeply concerned that *any perpetuation of the conflict over Oshin's treatment will continue to diminish the ability of his parents to focus their energies solely on the provision of that support and love directly to him when he needs it most.* Taking into account all the medical and other evidence, I conclude that it is in Oshin's best interests to move to palliative care.
>
> (*Kiszko 3*, at [84]) [emphasis added]

This meant that attempts at curative treatment stopped. Oshin passed away on 28 December 2016 (Young, 2016).

Issues in respect of mandated treatment for minors

Other cases that have come before the courts in respect of treatment for minors have involved opposition to treatment by both minors, including children just short of their 18th birthday (see, e.g., *X v Sydney Children's Hospitals Network*, 2013), and by their parents. As noted earlier, the reasons for such opposition have principally been religious ('the Jehovah's Witness cases', e.g., *B v Director-General, Social Welfare*, 1996; *Children, Youth and Women's Health Services Inc v YJL* (2010); *Hospital v T,* 2015), and antagonism to conventional medicine ('the complementary medicine cases', e.g., *Re Charlie Gard*, 2017; the Holloway litigation in New Zealand (Breen, 2006)). Until the Oshin Kiszko decisions the courts in Australia, and generally in the United Kingdom, Canada and New Zealand, had permitted treatment recommended by clinicians. When the children were mature, this constituted a difficult collision between autonomy of decision-making in respect of treatment for very ill children, generally with one form or another of cancer, and what clinicians regarded as forms of medical intervention with a sufficient prospect of clinical success. Frequently, such intervention has involved chemotherapy and the use of replacement blood products, as well as some amount of risk arising from the treatment provided to the child. When it has involved younger children, the conflict has been between what parents have asserted were their entitlements and obligations to make treatment decisions in relation to their children and the views of clinicians. On occasions, child protection authorities have also been in the background, given concerns about the consequences of withholding of treatment for the wellbeing of children in need to medical care. Nevertheless, in spite of the notion of Gillick competence – in which a child is regarded as having significant and growing levels of capacity to accept or decline medical treatment as they approach their age of majority – and in spite of the role of parents generally as decision-makers about the treatment to be given to non-Gillick-competent children, with few exceptions courts have permitted the treatment sought by clinicians (see, e.g., *Re JM (Child)*, 2015), and the potency of the child's voice has been limited.

The Kiszko decisions are distinguished by several factors. First, Oshin was not Gillick-competent; at the relevant times he was only five and six years of age. Secondly, the opposition to treatment for Oshin came from both of his parents. Part of what drove their stance was a mistrust of conventional medicine and an ideological commitment to forms of therapy that were not evidence-based but asserted to be organic, holistic and directed toward the experience of life, rather than being 'cure-driven'. Thirdly, in Oshin's case attempts to resolve the health issues and to reach a resolution that was mutually acceptable to clinicians and Oshin's parents failed, resulting in serial resort to litigation by the clinicians and the media by Oshin's parents. Fourthly, as in the *King* and *Gard* litigation in England, Oshin's parents mounted a substantial and highly publicised campaign through the media, utilising consultants to increase the pressure on the hospital and the courts to conform to their views (for the same phenomenon in the Charlie Gard case, see Freckelton, 2017).

Another feature that distinguished the Kiszko litigation was that the clinical case for chemotherapy treatment and also for radiotherapy treatment was not as strong as in many comparable cases. Partly this was caused by the fact that the court processes and court orders delayed the provision of treatment and reduced its potential efficacy to the point that, by September, the prospects of curative success had become very low. The passage of time, the experience of treatment, and the determination of doctors to attempt to assist Oshin through the provision of treatment polarised the general community and entrenched the parties in a dynamic of opposed views.

The Oshin Kiszko litigation raises the difficult issues of how likely to be efficacious a treatment must be and how low the risks of adverse consequences needs to be for courts to invoke their *parens patriae* jurisdiction to authorise such treatment in a child's best interests in spite of opposition from them and/or their parents. The approach of Chief Justice Thackray was to authorise chemotherapy, finding the prospects of the success of such treatment on both occasions to be sufficient to justify its being authorised in spite of vehement opposition from Oshin's parents. However, he took a different position in relation to radiotherapy after being satisfied on the basis of expert evidence that such treatment raised real risks of long-term adverse consequences to Oshin's wellbeing. A significant factor predisposing him not to override the parents' position by the time of the second phase of the litigation was that by then, at least in respect of the radiotherapy option, the parents enjoyed the qualified support of a suitably qualified and experienced paediatric oncologist. The position Chief Justice Thackray adopted was not so much an endorsement of the parents' opposition to conventional medicine as an acknowledgment that the evidence established a serious and real potential for deleterious consequences flowing from the proposed treatment. In short, the position of the parents – while the clinicians disagreed with it, and so would most parents – was not wholly unreasonable. By contrast, in the mental health context it has been held that:

> where the decision is thought to be affected by the very condition which requires treatment, less weight may be accorded the choice: see, e.g., *Re W* where the psychiatric evidence indicated that the young person's decision was affected by her anorexia nervosa.
> (*X v The Children's Hospitals Network*, 2013, at [63] per Justice of Appeal Basten)

Another distinctive aspect of the Family Court of Western Australia's decision-making was the influence of the intractability of the position of Oshin's parents, and the risk that if treatment that was increasingly vehemently opposed by Oshin's parents was permitted, the decision would expose Oshin to his parents' hostility and bitterness to the treatment, causing him 'even more psychological trauma' at a time when he needed harmony and uncompromised support. Thus, their position, by reason of being fixed, determined and 'irrational', was found to be such as to damage the already fragile state of their son, and thereby became a potent factor in whether life-saving treatment for him should be authorised by the court. It was in these circumstances that in spite of the urgency of a decision, Justice O'Brien reserved what became the final decision in the litigation for several days, noting that his reasons would set up 'a framework' for future cases (see McNeill & Young, 2016). What took place did not so much relate to the infliction of distress on Oshin directly by reason of the treatment but indirectly by reason of the distress caused to Oshin's parents and thus to him by the impairment of their capacity to look after him empathically. Generally, the emotional impact of coerced treatment is not overtly factored into the calculus of whether treatment, such as involuntary mental health treatment, should be ordered. However, in the context of a jurisdiction that explicitly incorporates a holistic determination of best interests, Chief Justice Thackray was significantly influenced by the indirect consequences for Oshin's emotional wellbeing that were likely to flow from the imposition of coercion.

The adversarialism into which Oshin Kiszko's case degenerated was a tragic example of what can sometimes be the failure of effective discourse or viable compromise in cases involving treatment for children's life-threatening illnesses. It is clearly preferable that such issues be resolved by non-litigious means, an aspiration also raised by Justice Francis in the Charlie Gard case in England (*Great Ormond Street Hospital v Yates*, 2017, at [131]). However, the courts function as a last resort to determine what is in the best interests of children in such situations (as also in cases involving persons with mental illnesses, brain injuries or intellectual disabilities). In Oshin's case a particularly difficult issue, on the basis of evolving evidence about the statistical prospects of his surviving his illness with or without chemotherapy or radiotherapy, was whether his parents' wish for him to be allowed to die with dignity and without intrusive interventions should be permitted to replace attempts at cure. Chief Justice Thackray and Justice O'Brien acknowledged that such a decision involves an attempt at rapprochement between profoundly opposing perspectives and that the issues are more than physical or medical – they are about the welfare of a child, which can be measured in multiple ways and must be evaluated in the particular context of his or her life. Chief Justice Thackray determined that a court should only overturn parental decisions about treatment of their child when there is clear justification to do so, and held that such justification does not exist where there is a clear medical opinion in favour of the parents' position, although that expert opinion may be a minority opinion. Whether a similar position obtains in relation to when the opposition to treatment comes from a Gillick-competent child is unclear.

The issue arises as to whether inherent in the evaluation of best interests are particular expectations by the courts as to the kind of life that people are expected to live – including, to use the words of Justice of Appeal Basten in *X v Children's Network Hospitals* (2013, at [73]) 'the state's interest in keeping a child alive not being jeopardised.' A related dilemma is the extent to which courts should use coercion to pursue every means at clinicians' disposal to preserve life in spite of what that may mean for quality of life, especially when the patient is a child. This was an important theme in the position Oshin's parents adopted. The reasoning of both Chief Justice Thackray and Justice O'Brien ultimately accepted that sanctity of life does not have a transcendent value, but when the courts will accept that emotional wellbeing and what is asserted to be the option of a 'dignified death' should trump a 'painful life' or the abandonment of hope for prolongation of life is not easily identified, especially in a jurisdiction in which 'best interests' have often been regarded as close to coterminous with adoption of all measures available for maintenance of life.

The Kiszko litigation constituted the reverse side of the coin to the subsequent high-profile Charlie Gard litigation in England (see Freckelton, 2017), which followed Charlie's parents raising £1.3 million through crowd funding to enable him to have access to speculative nucleoside therapy in the United States for a rare inherited disease known as mitochondrial DNA depletion syndrome. This option was opposed by Charlie's clinicians, who successfully sought orders to prevent the eight-month-old's removal to the United States. Justice Francis (*Great Ormond Street Hospital v Yates*, 2017) and then the Court of Appeal (*Yates v Greater Ormond Street Hospital*, 2017, at [39]), the Supreme Court and the European Court of Human Rights concluded that taking Charlie to the United States for such treatment would be futile and therefore contrary to his best interests. They determined that instead he should receive palliative care. In addition to the best interests consideration, Justice Francis (at [40]) also applied United Kingdom Supreme Court authority (*Aintree University Hospital NHS Foundation Trust v James*, 2013) that decision-makers:

> must try and put themselves in the place of the individual patient and ask what his attitude to the treatment is or would be likely to be; and they must consult others who are looking after him or interested in his welfare, in particular for their view of what his attitude would be.
>
> (at [39])

Charlie's independent legal representative did not support the proposed treatment, so it was through that source that there was investigation of what his attitude might be.

The unfortunate Kiszko saga illustrates the dangers when courts are asked to override either a mature minor's refusal of consent for potentially life-preserving medical treatment or when it is a non-Gillick-competent minor's parents who refuse to provide consent to clinician-recommended treatment. With the *parens patriae* jurisdiction focusing upon what is in the child's best interests, as well as the jurisdiction of the Family Court, the focus of a court's decision-making will be upon what in the overall context is determined to be in the child's best interests. Generally, the courts' approach has been to find that preserving the life of the child, even if this involves intrusive treatment or proceeding contrary to religious views or strong opinions about natural therapies, is in the child's best interests. However, as illustrated by the Kiszko decisions, the situation becomes more complex when the treatment may not be effective, when it may have seriously adverse consequences for the child, or where it may reduce the quality of the final phases of a very ill child's life. In such circumstances coercion of treatment may be experienced as oppressive or counter-therapeutic, and proceeding against the wishes of the child or the parents may ultimately be contrary to the best interests of the child. However, it is also problematic that certain decisions by courts or certain processes leading to such decisions may give a fillip to oppositionalism to treatment that is based on fixed ideological positions or even irrationality, however well intentioned.

This highlights the need to avoid the involvement of the courts and trial by media, wherever this can be done, by every available form of non-adversarial technique, as their involvement introduces aspects of conflict and notoriety which are contaminating, unhelpfully distracting and entrenching, and seldom therapeutic. In the Charlie Gard litigation, Justice Francis observed that a means of reducing the level of stand-off between parents and clinicians would have been:

> some form of Issues Resolution Hearing or other form of mediation where the parties can have confidential conversations to see what common ground can be reached between them. I believe that that type of hearing, be it Judge led or some other form of private mediation, would have led to a greater understanding between the parents and the clinical team in this case. I am not saying that it would necessarily have led to a resolution, but I think in many such cases it would and I would like to think that in future cases like this such attempts can be made.
>
> (*Yates v Greater Ormond Street Hospital*, 2017, at [130]; see too *Re Gard (A Child)*, 2017, at [20])

However, while it is trite, it remains true to observe that when courts are thrust into a decision-making role in life and death treatment scenarios, the decisions that have to be made are extraordinarily confronting and difficult for all concerned. In particular, balancing the relevant human rights and factoring the views of the child and of their parents into what objectively in the particular circumstances is in the child's best interests is particularly challenging. Inevitably it involves a range of value judgments, only some of which are likely to be explicitly articulated and many of which may be the subject of strongly held differences of opinion.

References

Adams, B. (2002, March 27). Australian girl flees to London to defy doctors. *New Zealand Herald*. www.nzherald.co.nz/world/news/article.cfm?c_id=2&objectid=1292036

Bacchi, C., & Beasley, C. (2002). Citizen bodies: is embodied citizenship a contradiction in terms? *Critical Social Policy* 22(2), 324–352.

Breen, C. (2006). *Age discrimination and children's rights: Ensuring equality and children's rights: Ensuring equality and acknowledging difference.* Amsterdam: Martinus Nijhoff Publishers.

Carter, B., Stickley, T., Inglis, S., & Laxon, A. (2002, June 6). Science, religion and a dying baby. *New Zealand Herald*. www.nzherald.co.nz/nz/news/article.cfm?c_id=1&objectid=2045181

Freckelton, I. (2016). Parents' opposition to potentially life-saving treatment for minors: learning from the Oshin Kiszko litigation. *Journal of Law and Medicine* 24, 61.

Freckelton, I., & McGregor, S. (2016). Refusal of potentially life-saving treatment for minors: The emerging international consensus by courts. *Journal of Law and Medicine* 23, 813.

Freckelton, I., & McGregor, S. (2017). Refusal of potentially life-saving treatment for minors. In I. Freckelton & K. Petersen (Eds.), *Tensions and traumas in health law*. Sydney: Federation Press.

Freckelton, I. (2017). Futility of treatment for dying children: Lessons from the Charlie Gard Litigation. *Journal of Law and Medicine* 25, 7.

Kallert, T.W., Mezzich, J.E., & Monahan, J. (Eds.) (2011). *Coercive treatment in psychiatry: Clinical, legal and ethical aspects*. Hoboken, NJ: Wiley-Blackwell.

MacLaughlin, S., Tolj, B., Huffadine, L., Eddie, R., & Noble, F. (2016, August 26). Doctors fighting in court to force a family to send their cancer-stricken son, six, for chemotherapy admit his chances of survival are 'remote'. *Daily Mail*. www.dailymail.co.uk/news/article-3759120/Perth-doctors-say-Oshin-Kiszko-s-chances-survival-remote-want-treatment-anyway.html

McNeill, H., & Young, E. (2016, August 25). 'This will set a precedent': Judge's decision for Oshin. *WA Today*. www.watoday.com.au/wa-news/this-will-set-a-precedent-judges-cancer-treatment-decision-for-oshin-20160825-gr16tx.html

Tyler, T.T. (1996). The psychological consequences of judicial procedures: Implications for civil commitment hearings. In D. Wexler & B. Winick (Eds.), *Law in a therapeutic key: Developments in therapeutic jurisprudence*. Durham, NJ: Carolina Academic Press.

Winick, B. J. (1997). Coercion and mental health treatment. *Denver Law Review* 74, 1145.

Young, E. (2016, December 30). The case of Oshin Kiszko: Think before you judge. *Sydney Morning Herald*. www.smh.com.au/comment/the-case-of-oshin-kiszko-think-before-you-judge-20161229-gtjjh8.html

Cases

Aintree University Hospital NHS Foundation Trust v. James [2013] UKSC 67
B v Director-General, Social Welfare [1996] 2 NZFR 134
CDJ v VAJ (1998) 197 CLR 172

Part IV

Paternalistic logics and their alternatives: interventions in 'vulnerability' and 'risk'

The previous three parts of this book raised difficult questions about the ongoing use of coercive interventions in society. Contributors to Part I considered whether coerced forms of treatment are supported by empirical evidence of their effectiveness. The answer to this question was not clear and ultimately is not simply an empirical one. As such, contributors to Part II engaged with this query from a different angle. Here it was asked if the inherently violent nature of these practices meant that regardless of how 'effective' these interventions prove to be, their significant material impacts and deleterious lived effects leaves them without foundation. For the contributors in this second part of the book, the resounding answer was 'yes'. And yet, as contributors in Part III argued, regardless of what we ultimately deem to be the most significant or telling effect of coercive interventions (their treatment efficiencies or deleterious lived effects), society may never choose to do away with these forced practices because they so neatly intersect with overarching and longstanding goals of governance and population management. Thus, this leaves us with one final question: how do we move forward from here? This is the focus in this final part of the book.

For John Chesterman of the Office of the Public Advocate, an answer to this question lies in our capacity to move beyond systems predicated on substitute decision-making principles. Chesterman's chapter on adult guardianship laws makes clear that if we want to succeed in significantly narrowing the use of powers that remove the decision-making authority of adults, then we need to ensure that a range of alternative measures are put in place to respond to situations in which these adults are asked to make important decisions about their lives, health and wellbeing. For Chesterman, this alternative vision comes in the form of supported decision-making processes that work in earnest to facilitate and not supplement the decisions of adults in need.

However, even in Chesterman's case, there is an acknowledgment that in certain situations of absolute necessity, some very limited form of substitute decision-making practices may be warranted. This acknowledgement raises the question: in such situations, is there a way to move forward to reduce the kinds of harms previously described in this book? Penelope Weller's chapter on compulsory mental health treatment offers one response.

In her chapter, Weller acknowledges that in mental health settings, difficult decisions sometimes need to be made about coercively intervening in the lives of adults who are very unwell. In these scenarios, Weller argues, some of the worst effects of coercive interventions can be ameliorated by applying therapeutic and procedurally just approaches to law; that is, approaches to law that recognise that the law and its decision-makers can have therapeutic (and harmful) effects, and approaches to law that recognise that the therapeutic effects of the law can be enhanced when decisions are made transparent in procedure. Accordingly, Weller argues that better outcomes could be achieved in mental health settings if the difficult decision about the need to coercively intervene in the life of an adult was made in a transparent, procedurally fair fashion, involving the adult in question being treated with dignity and respect. Yet this is only one imagined future offered in this final part of the book, and one which is not necessarily shared by other contributors.

In his chapter, Jamie Walvisch argues for the line between law and therapy to be redefined, such that the treatment needs of mentally ill offenders are decoupled from the communicative purposes of law's punishments. Walvisch argues that the current sentencing framework requires a radical reorganisation, and that sentencing should only ever focus on the communicative aims of punishment – repentance, reform and reconciliation – and not the consequentialist goals of deterrence, rehabilitation and community protection. He proposes that if we move towards this vision of 'communicative retributivism', then the situations in which a court could order offenders to seek mental health treatment as part of their sentences would be severely limited. Walvisch contends that even in these severely limited cases in which the court might find grounds to order an offender to seek mental health treatment, it would still be understood under this vision of 'communicative retributivism' that the offender remains a responsible moral agent who is allowed to refuse such treatment and opt for a different sanction of equal severity should he or she see fit. This, Walvisch argues, is how we maintain the autonomy, privacy and freedom of people with mental health concerns. This imagined future sits in contrast with the vision imagined by Bernadette McSherry.

Like Walvisch, McSherry's chapter engages with the question of what to do with offenders who have significant treatment needs, although in McSherry's case she is interested in one specific cohort: those who have already been imprisoned for serious offences and who are deemed at high risk of reoffending. McSherry acknowledges that this particular cohort is at risk of being subject to post-sentence detention and supervision regimes which effectively act as a form of double punishment. She argues that these approaches offend against human rights frameworks, and advocates for a form of mandated treatment that would better serve the needs of these individuals. Specifically, McSherry advocates for a coordinated response that would see these individuals subject to intensive case management which targets criminogenic and therapeutic needs, addressing the individual's accommodation, psycho-social and other needs. She argues that this approach to mandated treatment, while not ideal in its mandated (as opposed to voluntary) form, is ultimately more defensible than containment alone.

In these ways, these final four substantive chapters of this edited collection remind us that there is little consistency at this time amongst scholars and practitioners about the best ways to move beyond the harms of coercive interventions, and that there is significant scope for other ideas to be added to this mix.

Chapter 11

Mandated treatment as punishment

Exploring the second Verdins principle

Jamie Walvisch

> The problem of the mentally disordered offender raises in a particularly acute form the question of the primary function of the courts.
>
> (Wootton, 1963, p. 58)

People with mental health problems occupy a central place in the criminal justice system. Although it is difficult to know the precise proportion of offenders with such problems, it is clear that it is exceedingly high. For example, in 2008 the World Health Organization (2008) estimated that of the nine million prisoners worldwide, at least one million had a significant mental disorder, and even more had common mental health problems such as depression and anxiety. This appears to be a worldwide phenomenon which extends to both men and women (see, e.g., Fazel & Seewald, 2012).

While some offenders with mental health problems will be diverted away from the criminal justice system (see, e.g., James, 2010; Richardson & McSherry, 2010), and a very small number of others will be found unfit to plead or will be acquitted on the basis of the 'insanity' defence (or its jurisdictional equivalent) (see, e.g., Mackay et al., 2006; Mackay et al., 2007), the vast majority will stand trial in the traditional way, and will face the normal sentencing process. This raises the crucial question of how their mental health problems should be taken into account by a sentencing judge.

When addressing this issue, Australian courts initially focused on the conflict between the fact that mental health problems may reduce an offender's culpability (suggesting the need for a lesser penalty), but may also increase the danger he or she poses to the community (suggesting the need for an increased penalty) (see, e.g., *Channon v R* (1978) 20 ALR 1; *Veen v R [No.1]* (1979) 143 CLR 458). The courts have subsequently made it clear that there are other ways in which an offender's mental health problems may affect his or her sentence; for example, they can affect the weight a judge should give to the principle of general deterrence (see, e.g., *R v Engert* (1995) 84 A Crim R 67).

In 2007, in the landmark case of *R v Verdins* (2007, 16 VR 260), the Victorian Court of Appeal refined and expanded the principles relating to the sentencing of offenders with mental health problems. In that case, the Court identified six ways in which a 'mental disorder or abnormality or impairment of mental functioning' could affect sentencing:

1 by reducing the offender's moral culpability;
2 by influencing the kind of sentence to be imposed and the conditions in which it should be served;
3 by moderating or eliminating the need for general deterrence;
4 by moderating or eliminating the need for specific deterrence;
5 by making a sentence weigh more heavily on the offender than on a person in normal health; or
6 by creating a serious risk of imprisonment having a significant adverse effect on the offender's mental health.

These 'Verdins principles' were subsequently adopted in all other Australian jurisdictions, as well as in New Zealand (see Walvisch, 2010, for case citations).

Although the Verdins principles have been discussed in over 500 higher court decisions in Victoria since 2007, as well as in academic papers (see, e.g., Freckelton, 2007; Gee, 2014; Walvisch, 2010), there has been very little discussion of the second Verdins principle: the fact that an offender's mental health problems can affect the *kind of sentence* to be imposed and its conditions. I seek to address that gap in this chapter, focusing in particular on the issue of mandated mental health treatment. The chapter starts by explaining the circumstances in which Victorian courts have held that an offender's mental health problems should affect the kind of sentence to be imposed, and the conditions in which it should be served. It then examines two different notions of capacity that are implicit in the courts' approach to this issue. Following that, the chapter looks at the courts' justification for mandating mental health treatment, before critiquing that justification on the basis that it denies offenders' autonomy. The chapter concludes by suggesting a revised approach to the second Verdins principle.

The current approach to the second Verdins principle

To date, there appear to have been five different ways in which an offender's mental health problems have influenced the kind of sentence that has been imposed, or the conditions in which it should be served, in the superior courts.[1] First, in rare cases the court has ordered that the offender serve his or her term of imprisonment in a mental health facility rather than a prison. This kind of order – known as a 'court secure treatment order' (formerly a 'hospital security order') – may only be made if:

i the offender would ordinarily have been sentenced to a term of imprisonment;

ii the court has considered the offender's current mental condition, medical history, mental health history, forensic history and social circumstances;

iii the offender has been examined by a psychiatrist;

iv the court is satisfied that the offender has a mental illness, and because of that illness the offender needs treatment to prevent his or her mental or physical health seriously deteriorating, or serious harm being caused to the offender or another person;

v the offender will receive such treatment if he or she is made subject to the order;

vi there is no less restrictive means reasonably available to enable the offender to receive the necessary treatment; and

vii the court has received a report from the authorised psychiatrist of a relevant mental health service recommending that the order be made, and stating that there are facilities or services available for the detention and treatment of the offender. (*Sentencing Act 1991* (Vic) ss. 94A-94C).

Due to the onerous nature of these requirements, and the lack of available facilities and services, this option has only been exercised in two superior court cases since 2007: *R v Fitchett* [2008] VSC 258 and *R v Imadonmwonyi* [2008] VSCA 135.

Secondly, the court has occasionally mandated mental health treatment as part of the sentencing disposition. For the first seven years after the *Verdins* decision was handed down, there was only one superior court case in which such treatment was ordered: *R v Elias* [2013] VSC 123. The limited use of this sentencing option was likely due to the fact that there was no sentencing disposition which specifically provided for such treatment. However, in early 2012 a new sentencing disposition was introduced into Victoria: the Community Correction Order (CCO). As part of this order, the court may attach a condition that requires an offender to undergo a mental health assessment and treatment (*Sentencing Act 1991* (Vic) s. 48D(3)(e)). Such a condition has been imposed in more than 10 superior court cases since 2014 (see, e.g., *Ashweirth v R* [2015] VSCA 224).

Thirdly, an offender's mental health problems have occasionally been held to change the normal balance between the parole and non-parole periods. For example, when an offender has been diagnosed with mental health problems, the court has sometimes set a shorter than usual non-parole period (see, e.g., *Director of Public Prosecutions v Hosking* [2009] VSC 549; *Gray v R* [2010] VSCA 312). This option has been viewed as desirable when treatment of the offender's mental health problems cannot be properly undertaken in the prison environment. It is seen to allow treatment to be carried out in a timely manner, reducing the risk of the offender's mental health deteriorating while in prison. It also allows the offender's mental health problems to be monitored by the relevant authorities for a longer period of time once he or she is returned to the community, reducing the risk of reoffending.

Fourthly, there have been a few cases in which, due to an offender's mental health problems, the court has ordered a non-custodial sentence when a term of imprisonment would normally have been imposed. For example, in *Hancock v R* [2013] VSCA 199, the offender committed numerous armed robberies and attempted burglaries, which would ordinarily have led to a lengthy term of imprisonment. However, as she was pregnant and had been diagnosed with depression, she was instead given a CCO.

Finally, there have been cases in which the court has decided to suspend an offender's sentence in light of his or her mental health problems.[2] For example, in *R v Bernstein* [2008] VSC 254 the offender was an elderly lawyer who embezzled money from his partner and some of his clients. By the time of sentencing he had been diagnosed with an anxiety disorder. While the sentencing judge would ordinarily have imposed a lengthy sentence in such circumstances, in light of the offender's mental health condition and age he imposed a shorter sentence in conjunction with a fine. He also wholly suspended the offender's sentence, when he would not have done so otherwise.

Two notions of capacity implicit in the courts' approach

Two key themes can be discerned from the limited jurisprudence on the second *Verdins* principle. First, there appears to be a concern with the offender's *capacity to appropriately manage his or her mental health*. If an offender is considered to have diminished capacity to look after his or her own mental health, the court considers it justifiable to intervene – by hospitalising him or her, mandating treatment, or imposing a shorter than usual non-parole period.

A clear example of this concern can be seen in the case of *R v Elius* [2013] VSC 123. In that case the offender was a 44-year-old woman who had been diagnosed with severe depression (at times of psychotic proportions), severe anxiety and benzodiazepine dependence. She devised a plan to win back custody of her daughter (who had been removed from her due to concerns over her abuse of alcohol) by having her ex-husband and his second wife disabled, hiring an undercover police officer to undertake the assault. She was convicted of incitement to cause serious injury. The sentencing judge was satisfied that her actions were a consequence of her mental health problems, and that if she received psychiatric care her chances of reoffending were negligible. Consequently, he released her on a six-month undertaking to place herself in the care of her psychiatrist, comply with all of his lawful and reasonable directions for her psychiatric treatment, and be of good behaviour. He explained his decision to mandate treatment to the offender in the following terms:

> I remain concerned that you are in need of continuing psychiatric care and that, without some form of compulsion or at least external discipline, you

might fail to ensure that you get it or comply with the recommendations of those who treat you.

(*R v Elias* [2013] VSC 123, [27])

The second theme that can be discerned from the cases is a concern with the offender's *capacity to cope with the travails of imprisonment*. When an offender is seen to be likely to have difficulties coping with prison due to his or her mental health problems, the court considers it justifiable to impose a non-custodial sanction. This can be seen in the cases of *Hancock v R* [2013] VSCA 199 and *R v Bernstein* [2008] VSC 254 discussed above. In *Hancock*, the court noted that it was taking the unusual step of imposing a CCO (rather than a prison sentence) because the offender's depression and pregnancy would make prison more onerous for her, and may have a detrimental effect on her mental health ([37]–[38]). In *Bernstein*, Judge of Appeal Nettle explained to the offender that the purpose of suspending his sentence was 'to avoid subjecting a man of your age and health to the rigour of gaol' ([57]).

There are difficulties with both of these concepts of capacity, which use paternalist and protectionist logics to sustain the use of coercive and intrusive medico-legal interventions (see Hannah-Moffat & Maurutto, 2012; Spivakovsky & Seear, 2017). Unfortunately, I do not have the scope to address them both in detail in this chapter. Consequently, the remainder of this chapter will focus solely on the first theme: the offender's capacity to appropriately manage his or her mental health.

Mandated treatment as punishment: the current approach

At first glance, it may not seem obvious why a sentencing judge, whose primary function is to impose punishment on offenders, may consider it appropriate to mandate mental health treatment for an offender who cannot manage his or her mental health. How can *treatment* be a form of *punishment*?

The answer to this question lies in the hybrid nature of the Victorian sentencing system.[3] While it is correct to say that the sentencing process is inherently punitive, punishment is not the only purpose a sentencing judge may try to achieve. Under section 5(1) of the *Sentencing Act 1991* (Vic), a judge may also impose a sentence for the purposes of deterrence, rehabilitation, denunciation or community protection. Thus, a judge may permissibly mandate treatment if that would help achieve any of these purposes.

The goal of community protection seems to underlie many of the courts' decisions to order a mental health treatment condition as part of a CCO. The courts' reasoning in these cases appears to be: the offender is unable to properly manage his or her own mental health; as a result, he or she poses a risk to others; it is therefore necessary to impose a mental health treatment condition in order to reduce that risk. This can be clearly seen in the case of

Director of Public Prosecutions v Maxfield [2015] VSCA 95, in which the sentencing judge:

> had regard to Ms Maxfield's intellectual disability and psychological difficulties, and concluded that the objective of community protection was more likely to be achieved – through the reduction of the risk of reoffending – by [imposing a CCO] with appropriate conditions attached, rather than by imposing a prison sentence.
>
> ([34])

The concern for community protection is often intertwined with a concern for rehabilitation, with mental health treatment mandated both because it protects others and is seen to be in the offender's own interests (since he or she cannot appropriately manage his or her own mental health). This approach can be seen in *R v Rose* [2015] VSC 614, a case in which an elderly offender who was diagnosed with various mental health problems (including delusional disorder, depressive disorder and an acquired brain injury) was convicted of intentionally causing serious injury (due to assaulting a co-resident at his aged care facility). When imposing a five-year CCO, with a mental health treatment condition, the judge told Mr Rose that the length and nature of the order 'reflects the seriousness of your offence and the need to deter and rehabilitate you, not only in your interests, but in the interests of the protection of the community, in particular your immediate community at McLellan House' ([56]).

This concern for both the community's and the offender's interests can also be clearly seen in *Ivanoff v R* [2015] VSCA 262, a case in which the offender, who was diagnosed with a major depressive disorder, was convicted of cultivating a commercial quantity of cannabis. The sentencing judge explained the reasons for imposing the CCO on the offender in the following terms:

> The idea is that I intend to deter you and others from engaging in the conduct you did, but also encourage your rehabilitation with extended time on a community corrections order. Both you and the community benefit while you are supported in your depression, and it is hoped that you will not reoffend.
>
> ([21])

The courts' approach to this issue could be critiqued on several grounds. For example, it is unclear precisely when an offender should be considered sufficiently incapable of managing his or her mental health that such intervention is justified: how much of a risk does he or she need to pose to him or herself or others? It is also unclear what limits (if any) should be imposed on the courts' ability to order mental health treatment. For example, would it be acceptable to order electroconvulsive therapy (ECT) or psychosurgery if those techniques would help to 'rehabilitate' the offender or make the community safer? From a broader perspective, the use of offenders' mental health problems to justify 'intensive, medico-legal interventions into the lives of subjects that are often already marginalized and stigmatized' may also be considered troubling (Spivakovsky & Seear, 2017, p. 466). However, in the remainder of this chapter I want to focus on one key issue: the courts' denial of offenders' autonomy.

Upholding offenders' autonomy in sentencing

In their guideline judgment on CCOs, the Victorian Court of Appeal lauded the CCO as a sentencing option which 'demands of the offender that he/she take personal responsibility for self-management and self-control' (*Boulton v R* [2014] VSCA 342, [114]). However, when a CCO is combined with a mental health treatment condition, this benefit of self-management fades away. Rather than providing offenders with the opportunity to seek treatment and thereby help themselves (and the community), their perceived lack of capacity to manage their own mental health provides grounds for the court to step in and force them to undergo treatment. In doing so, the court fails to treat offenders as autonomous agents, and instead draws on a paternalist and protectionist logic to intervene.

While those who adhere to a utilitarian philosophy of state may consider such a measure to be justified if it will enhance community safety (Munetz, Galon & Frese, 2003), I agree with Duff (1986) that civic society should be defined and structured by a shared commitment to autonomy, freedom and privacy. The state should uphold the community's defining values, treating all citizens (including offenders) in a way that respects those values (Duff, 2001). Consequently, if there is a desire to change people's behaviour for some reason, this should only be done by providing them with the relevant reasons for making such a change, and trying to persuade them to reform themselves (Duff, 1986).[4] It should be up to the individuals, as autonomous agents, whether or not to implement the recommended change.

If this commitment to autonomy is taken seriously, the sentencing system should not be seeking to achieve the consequentialist goals of deterrence, rehabilitation and community protection. To do so is to use people as a means to an end, rather than as an end in themselves. Instead, the primary purpose of punishment should be to communicate to offenders the censure they deserve for having committed a crime (see, e.g., Duff, 2001; Tadros, 2005; Von Hirsch & Ashworth, 2005). Such censure makes it clear that the conduct was wrong and is taken seriously by the state. It is hoped that by communicating this censure to offenders, they will be brought to recognise that they have acted wrongly, repent their crimes, reform their behaviour and be reconciled with the community (Duff, 2001).

On this account, with its emphasis on repentance, reform and reconciliation, punishment is seen to be a two-way process in which the state attempts to communicate with offenders, rather than a one-way expression of condemnation by the state (Duff, 1996). Duff considers this type of 'communicative retributivism' to be appropriate because it treats offenders as rational moral agents. It does so by appealing to their reason and understanding, and seeking a specific response from them (repentance and reform), rather than by simply imposing penalties on passive subjects (Duff, 1998). While offenders should not be forced to accept the state's censure as justified, it is hoped that they will understand and accept that they have been found to have committed a public wrong for which they are being properly censured, and to reform their behaviour accordingly (Duff, 2011).

It is important to note that the concept of 'reform' on which Duff relies is one of 'self-reform': punishment should seek to 'persuade offenders that and why they should reform themselves' (Duff, 2001, p. 91). This can be contrasted with a crude consequentialist concept of 'reform', which seeks to modify offenders' attitudes and behaviours in any way that will make them compliant with the law. Such a view fails to treat offenders as moral agents, instead treating them as objects to be moulded into whatever shape society considers desirable.

On this view of punishment, sentencing judges should move beyond traditional paternalist and protectionist logics, and should not require offenders to undergo mental health treatment for the purposes of rehabilitation or community protection, regardless of their (in)capacity to manage their own mental health. However, there are limited circumstances in which an offender's mental health problems should be taken into account in determining the kind of sentence to be imposed. These circumstances are discussed below.

A revised approach to the second Verdins principle

Under Duff's theory of punishment, the sentencing determination should be guided by the principle of negative proportionality (Duff, 2001, p. 143). Such a principle sets the outer boundaries of punishment: it holds that a sanction must not be disproportionately lenient or disproportionately severe. However, within those boundaries a sentencer has the flexibility to determine an appropriate sanction.

In some cases it will be clear what type of sanction should be imposed. For example, when the offender has committed a particularly serious crime, it may be the case that the only type of punishment that can express a sufficient amount of censure is imprisonment. However, in other cases there may be two (or more) types of sanction that would be proportionate to the offence. For example, it may be the case that either a short period of imprisonment or a CCO would be appropriate. In such cases, Duff (2001) argues that the selection of the proper sanction should be determined by the communicative purposes of punishment. That is, the sentencer should impose a sanction that not only conveys an appropriate level of censure, but also helps achieve the goals of repentance, reform and reconciliation. Duff suggests that this can best be achieved by imposing a sanction that displays a substantive understanding of the particular crime and its implications.

In the sections below I examine two types of case in which an offender's mental health problems may affect the sentencer's selection of the proper sanction: those in which the offender's mental health problems substantially contributed to the offence; and those in which the communicative aims of punishment would be better served by one of the available sanctions. While these categories are independent, they are not mutually exclusive.

Mental health problems that substantially contributed to the offence

When an offender's mental health problems substantially contributed to the offence in some way, it may be appropriate for the sentencer to fashion a sentence that makes that fact clear, thereby demonstrating a substantive understanding of the offence. For example, if the sentencer finds that the offender's depression substantially contributed to the offence, he or she could require the offender to seek treatment for that depression as part of his or her sentence. Such a requirement would make it clear that, in the sentencer's view, there was a significant link between the depression and the offending behaviour. Receiving such treatment may also help the offender repent his or her wrongdoing, reform his or her behaviour and become reconciled with the community.

In this context, the sentencer may take into account *any* mental health problems that substantially contributed to the offending behaviour, regardless of their cause or nature. However, it is necessary for the sentencer to find that the offender's mental health problems *substantially* contributed to the offending behaviour before taking them into account in fashioning a sanction. This is because a sentence which focused on the offender's mental health problems in the absence of a substantial contribution would falsely imply that those problems were integral to the offence. Such a sentence would not convey a substantive understanding of the offence.

Determining whether the offender's mental health problems substantially contributed to the offence is a legal issue, not a psychiatric one. Evidence should be targeted at the offender's mental functioning at the time of the offence, not simply on the existence of a diagnosed disorder. Expert witnesses should focus on the specific ways in which the offender's mental health problems *may* have contributed to the offending behaviour: it should not be assumed that merely because the offender has been diagnosed with a mental health problem, there must be a link. It is for the sentencer to decide whether the offender's mental health problem *did* contribute to the offence, and whether this should influence the choice of available sanctions.

Care needs to be taken to ensure that any conditions imposed on the offender treat him or her as a responsible moral agent, and still attempt to solicit a repentant understanding of the offence through punishment. This has three important consequences. First, offenders should be free to reject mental health treatment conditions, opting instead for equally serious but less intrusive sanctions. Secondly, sentencers should not require offenders to take medication or undergo psycho-surgery as a means of reforming their behaviour. Such measures try to side-step the necessary process of punishment, and do not address offenders as responsible moral agents (Duff, 1986). Thirdly, sentencers should not require offenders to serve their sentences in a hospital or mental health treatment facility. Given their treatment focus, such institutions are not well suited to achieving the communicative aims of punishment.

I do not intend to suggest that offenders who are unwell, and who require medical assistance, should be denied that help. It is essential that offenders continue to be treated as citizens, and this includes providing them with the same level of medical care as other citizens. However, the treatment needs of offenders differ from the communicative purposes that must be served when determining the appropriate mode of punishment, and should be kept separate.

Mental health problems that affect the communicative aims of punishment

The other circumstance in which an offender's mental health problems may affect the kind of punishment which should be imposed occurs when the sentencer is satisfied that, due to the offender's mental health problems, the communicative aims of punishment would be better served by one of the available sanctions. This type of case can best be explained via an illustration. Imagine a case in which:

- the offender has been convicted of his second assault, for which an appropriate sanction is either a short term of imprisonment or a lengthy period of home detention;
- the sentencer is of the view that the offender's mental health problems contributed to his offending behaviour;
- the sentencer is of the view that the goals of repentance and reform will be best served if the offender receives treatment for his mental health problems; and
- treatment for the offender's mental health problems is only available outside prison.

In such circumstances, it would be appropriate for the sentencer to select home detention as the sanction to impose, as that sanction is best likely to serve the communicative purposes of punishment.

The mental health problems that are relevant in this context differ from those discussed above. In this context, any mental health problems which are likely to affect the communicative aims of punishment may be relevant, even if those mental health problems did not contribute to the offending behaviour in any way. Once again, this is a legal issue not a psychiatric one. Consequently, expert evidence should be targeted at the effects of the offender's mental health problems, not the existence of a specific disorder. Expert witnesses should focus on the ways in which the offender's mental health problems may affect the processes of repentance and self-reform under each of the available sanctions. It is for the sentencer to decide whether the mental health problems are likely to affect the communicative purposes of those sanctions, and whether that should influence the sentencing disposition.

It is important to note that I am not suggesting that the offender's sentence should be reduced on this basis. The offender's mental health problems simply provide a reason for choosing between equally severe sanctions. Thus, in the example provided above, the sentencer did not select home detention because it was a less severe sanction than imprisonment. Similarly, the sentencer could not have imposed home detention if such a sanction was not considered sufficiently severe for an offence as serious as that committed by the offender. This is in contrast to the approach Victorian courts currently take to the second *Verdins* principle. Under that approach, the principle is sometimes used as the basis for imposing a less severe sanction on the offender (see, e.g., *Hancock v R* [2013] VSCA 199; *R v Bernstein* [2008] VSC 254).

Conclusion

The epigraph at the beginning of this chapter notes that offenders with mental health problems raise, in a particularly acute form, the question of the primary function of the courts. I have suggested in this chapter that sentencing courts should move beyond paternalistic and protectionist logics, and instead be guided by the fundamental principles of autonomy, freedom and privacy. Their primary function should be to communicate to offenders the censure they deserve for having committed a crime. It is hoped that by doing so, offenders will come to repent their crimes, reform their behaviour and be reconciled with the community.

Under such an approach, it would not be appropriate for sentencers to require offenders to undergo mental health treatment against their will, simply because they are seen to be incapable of managing their own mental health. Similarly, it would not be permissible to order an offender to serve his or her sentence in a hospital rather than a prison. Such dispositions undermine offenders' autonomy and are incompatible with the communicative purposes of punishment.

However, there are two circumstances in which an offender's mental health problems may affect the kind of sentence that should be imposed or its conditions: cases in which the offender's mental health problems substantially contributed to the offence; and cases in which the communicative aims of punishment would be better served by one of the available sanctions. In such cases, it may be appropriate for a court to order an offender to seek mental health treatment. However, it is essential that offenders are always treated as responsible moral agents, and are allowed to refuse such treatment and opt for a different sanction of equal severity.

While this approach would require a radical reorganisation of the current sentencing framework, replacing the consequentialist principles of deterrence, rehabilitation and community protection with a form of communicative retributivism, this is necessary to protect the autonomy of some of the most marginalised citizens in our society – offenders with mental health problems.

Notes

1 This typology is based on an analysis of the 537 Victorian Supreme Court and Court of Appeal cases in which the *Verdins* decision was raised between 23 May 2007 (when the decision was handed down) and 31 July 2016. It is possible that an offender's mental health problems have affected the kind of sentence that has been imposed in other ways in the lower courts (the County Court and the Magistrates' Court).
2 The ability to suspend a sentence was abolished in Victoria from 1 September 2014: see *Sentencing Amendment (Abolition of Suspended Sentences and Other Matters) Act 2013* (Vic).
3 All Australian sentencing systems of are of a similarly hybrid nature, as are the sentencing systems in Canada and the United Kingdom: see *Criminal Code* (Can), RSC 1985, c C-46, s. 718; *Criminal Justice Act 2003* (UK) c 44, s. 142.
4 It is important to note that my focus is on the sentencing context, and that individuals who face the sentencing process are assumed to be rational moral agents. If, due to their mental health problems, they were either incapable of recognising and responding to the reasons that bore on their situation at the time of the offence, or cannot properly engage in the trial process, they should be acquitted on the grounds of a defence such as 'insanity' or found unfit to plea or stand trial (see Duff, 2007).

References

Duff, R. A. (1986). *Trials and punishment*. Cambridge: Cambridge University Press.
Duff, R. A. (1996). Punishment, citizenship and responsibility. In H. Tam (Ed.), *Punishment, excuses and moral development* (pp. 17–34). Farnham: Ashgate Publishing.
Duff, R. A. (1998). Punishment, communication, and community. In M. Matravers (Ed.), *Punishment and political theory* (pp. 48–68). Oxford: Hart Publishing.
Duff, R. A. (2001). *Punishment, communication, and community*. Oxford: Oxford University Press.
Duff, R. A. (2007). *Answering for crime: Responsibility and liability in the criminal law*. Oxford: Oxford University Press.
Duff, R. A. (2011). Good and evil and the criminal law. In C. Cordner (Ed.), *Philosophy, ethics and a common humanity: Essays in honour of Raymond Gaita* (pp. 68–81). New York: Routledge.

Fazel, S., & Seewald, K. (2012). Severe mental illness in 33,588 prisoners worldwide: Systematic review and meta-regression analysis. *British Journal of Psychiatry* 200, 364–373.

Freckelton, I. (2007). Sentencing offenders with impaired mental functioning. *Psychiatry, Psychology and Law* 14, 359–363.

Gee, D. (2014). Sentencing offenders with impaired mental functioning: R v Verdins, Buckley and Vo [2007] at the clinical coalface. *Psychiatry, Psychology and Law* 21, 46–66.

Hannah-Moffat, K., & Maurutto, P. (2012). Shifting and targeted forms of penal governance: bail, punishment and specialized courts. *Theoretical Criminology* 13, 201–219.

James, D. V. (2010). Diversion of mentally disordered people from the criminal justice system in England and Wales: An overview. *International Journal of Law and Psychiatry* 33, 241–248.

Mackay, R. D., Mitchell, B. J., & Howe, L. (2006). Yet more facts about the insanity defence. *Criminal Law Review*, 399–411.

Mackay, R. D., Mitchell, B. J., & Howe, L. (2007). A continued upturn in unfitness to plead – more disability in relation to the trial under the 1991 Act. *Criminal Law Review*, 530–544.

Munetz, M. R., Galon, P. A., & Frese, F. J. (2003). The ethics of mandatory community treatment. *Journal of the American Academy of Psychiatry and Law* 31, 173–183.

Richardson, E., & McSherry, B. (2010). Diversion down under – programs for offenders with mental illnesses in Australia. *International Journal of Law and Psychiatry* 33, 249–257.

Spivakovsky, C., & Seear, K. (2017). Making the abject: Problem-solving courts, addiction, mental illness and impairment. *Continuum* 31, 458–469.

Tadros, V. (2005). *Criminal responsibility.* Oxford: Oxford University Press.

Von Hirsch, A., & Ashworth, A. (2005). *Proportionate sentencing: exploring the principles.* Oxford: Oxford University Press.

Walvisch, J. (2010). Sentencing offenders with impaired mental functioning: Developing Australia's 'most sophisticated and subtle' analysis. *Psychiatry, Psychology and Law* 17, 187–201.

Wootton, B. (1963). *Crime and the criminal law: reflections of a magistrate and social scientist.* London: Stevens and Sons.

World Health Organization (2008). *Trenčín statement on prisons and mental health.* Geneva: WHO.

Cases

Ashweirth v R [2015] VSCA 224.
Boulton v R [2014] VSCA 342.
Channon v R (1978) 20 ALR 1.
Director of Public Prosecutions v Hosking [2009] VSC 549.
Director of Public Prosecutions v Maxfield [2015] VSCA 95.
Gray v R [2010] VSCA 312.
Hancock v R [2013] VSCA 199.
Ivanoff v R [2015] VSCA 262.

R v Bernstein [2008] VSC 254.
R v Elias [2013] VSC 123.
R v Engert (1995) 84 A Crim R 67.
R v Fitchett [2008] VSC 258.
R v Imadonmwonyi [2008] VSCA 135.
R v Rose [2015] VSC 614.
R v Verdins (2007) 16 VR 269.
Veen v R [No.1] (1979) 143 CLR 458.

Legislation

Sentencing Act 1991 (Vic).
Sentencing Amendment (Abolition of Suspended Sentences and Other Matters) Act 2013 (Vic).
Criminal Code (Can), RSC 1985, c C-46.
Criminal Justice Act 2003 (UK) c 44, s 142.

Chapter 12

Containment versus rehabilitation

Managing high-risk offenders with complex needs

Bernadette McSherry

Some individuals considered to be at high risk of serious offending display problem behaviours that need careful management. They can be viewed as members of a group of individuals with multiple and complex needs, which Margaret Hamilton (2010) has defined as including those 'who experience various combinations of mental illness, intellectual disability, acquired brain injury, physical disability, behavioural difficulties, homelessness, social isolation, family dysfunction and drug and/or alcohol misuse' (p. 307).

In recent years, schemes across Australia have been weighted in favour of the containment of such individuals through a variety of means, from control orders to post-sentence detention and supervision. One of the central justifications for containment schemes is that removing those considered to be at high risk of serious offending from the community, or at the very least intensively monitoring them, is the best way to stop them from harming others. These schemes may be viewed as being on a continuum from pre-crime to post-sentence detention. They encompass detention of suspected terrorists without charge and accused persons held on remand, as well as indefinite detention of high-risk recidivist offenders and post-sentence detention of sex offenders (McSherry, 2014).

Such schemes are not new. The term 'preventive justice' was first used in the late 18th century and linked to laws aimed at preventing future crime by intervening where there was a 'probable suspicion, that some crime is intended or likely to happen' (Blackstone, 1772). What is new is the emphasis placed on assessing the risk of future harmful behaviour. While there has been considerable criticism of the use of risk assessment instruments in this regard (McSherry, 2014), 'structured professional judgment', which combines statistical or actuarial risk prediction with clinical methods, has become an accepted way to identify those who are at low, moderate or high risk of harming others (Davis & Ogloff, 2008).

In this chapter I consider management and treatment options for a subgroup of such individuals: those who have been imprisoned for serious offences and who are deemed at high risk of reoffending. I argue that the coordination of services, together with the provision of treatment in the community, provides a better means of protecting the community than detention in institutions.

Containment options

In Australia, various legislative regimes are aimed at containing and controlling individuals considered to be at risk of serious offending. These include criminal justice schemes enabling indefinite sentences of serious offenders and civil justice schemes enabling post-sentence detention and supervision, primarily of sex offenders (Keyzer & McSherry, 2015; McSherry, 2014; McSherry & Keyzer, 2009; McSherry & Keyzer, 2011; McSherry, 2005). There are also preventive detention schemes for those who have not offended but are considered at risk of harming others, such as suspected terrorists and those with severe mental health problems (McSherry, 2014; McSherry, 2017). Some civil schemes that enable the detention of those with intellectual disabilities, severe mental health problems and/or substance abuse problems may be couched in terms of treatment, but the risk of harm to self or others usually forms part of the criteria for admission to a facility (McSherry, 2017). The common thread running through containment schemes is that they are predominantly aimed at community protection.

Individuals who have been found unfit to plead or not guilty on the grounds of mental impairment may also be indefinitely detained on this basis. While the unfitness to stand trial doctrine was largely incorporated into modern law as a humanistic measure to protect accused persons with disabilities from trials in which they are unable to participate, in practice, such persons can be detained for longer than if they had been convicted and sentenced following trial (Gooding et al., 2017). Marlon James Noble, for example, was detained in prison for nearly a decade after he was found unfit to stand trial in Western Australia in relation to alleged sexual assaults (Gooding et al., 2017). This was despite one of the alleged victims informing prosecutors Mr Noble had never assaulted them (Egan, 2011).

In relation to the sentencing process, the power to pass an indefinite sentence on offenders who are assessed as posing a danger to society exists in the Northern Territory (*Sentencing Act 1995* s 65), Queensland (*Penalties and Sentences Act 1992* s 163), Tasmania (*Sentencing Act 1997* s 19), Victoria (*Sentencing Act 1991* s 18A) and Western Australia (*Sentencing Act 1995* s 98). Some of these provisions specifically refer to violent offenders and sex offenders, while others are broader in their scope. In addition, Queensland (*Criminal Law Amendment Act 1945* s 18(1)–(3)) and South Australia (*Criminal Law (Sentencing) Act 1998* s 23) have special indefinite detention schemes for sex offenders that enable the relevant Attorney-General to apply for an order for continuing detention during the term of imprisonment.

Post-sentence detention and supervision of certain offenders has been initiated in many Australian jurisdictions and it seems there are no signs of it abating. In 2003, Queensland introduced a new scheme for post-sentence detention in prison and continuing supervision of sex offenders (*Dangerous Prisoners (Sexual Offenders) Act 2003*). Western Australia (*Dangerous Sexual Offenders Act 2006*), New South Wales (*Crimes (High Risk Offenders) Act 2006*), Victoria (*Serious Sex Offenders (Detention and Supervision) Act 2009*) and the Northern Territory (*Serious Sex Offenders Act 2013*) followed. The New South Wales legislation has been amended by the *Crimes (Serious Sex Offenders) Amendment Act 2013* (NSW), such that it now relates to 'high risk sex offenders and high risk violent offenders' (Sch 1, ss 1 and 3), but the main features of the scheme remain the same. A recent review of the regime in Victoria by the Complex Adult Victim Sex Offender Management Review Panel (2015) has also recommended that the scheme be altered to target those posing an unacceptable risk of serious interpersonal violence. The federal, state and territory governments have also announced through the Council of Australian Governments that they plan to pass legislation to enable the post-sentence preventive detention of those convicted of terrorism related offences (Smith & Nolan, 2016, p. 164).

These schemes pose significant human rights concerns. Human rights are considered rights inherent to all human beings, regardless of status. As described by Michael Brett Young (2015), they are '[t]he basic rights that belong to everyone, regardless of age, race, sex, or disability, income or education. They are about treating people fairly and with dignity, and ensuring individual rights are respected' (p. 3).

Some human rights are considered absolute, while others may be subject to reasonable limitations. For example, Article 9(1) of the *International Covenant on Civil and Political Rights* states that:

> Everyone has the right to liberty and security of person. No one shall be subjected to arbitrary arrest or detention. No one shall be deprived of his [or her] liberty except on such grounds and in accordance with such procedure as are established by law.

The wording of Article 9(1) indicates that there may be instances where the right to liberty can be subject to reasonable limitations. Article 14 of the United Nations *Convention on the Rights of Persons with Disabilities* (which as per its Article 1 applies to individuals with 'mental' and 'intellectual impairments' as well as physical disabilities) reiterates the right to liberty and security of the person.

Eleven of the 13 members of the United Nations Human Rights Committee have agreed that the New South Wales (*Re Tillman v Australia*) and Queensland (*Re Fardon v Australia*) schemes enabling post-sentence detention of sex offenders violate the right to liberty (McSherry, 2014, pp. 180–182 and references therein). They found that 'continued imprisonment or even detention' amounted to a fresh term of imprisonment, which was not permissible in the absence of a criminal conviction; it was viewed as a form of 'double punishment'. This position aligns with Justice Kirby's dissenting judgment in the High Court of Australia's *Fardon v Attorney-General (Qld)* decision, in which he observed (at 647) that:

> In Australia … punishment is reserved to courts in respect of the crimes that prisoners are proved to have committed. It is not available for crimes that are feared, anticipated or predicted to occur in the future on evidence that is notoriously unreliable and otherwise would be inadmissible and by people who do not have the gift of prophesy.

The Committee on the Rights of Persons with Disabilities (2015) also stated that

> [t]he involuntary detention of persons with disabilities based on risk or dangerousness, alleged need of care or treatment or other reasons tied to impairment or health diagnosis is contrary to the right to liberty, and amounts to arbitrary deprivation of liberty.
>
> (para. 13)

In response to the Human Rights Committee's findings, the Australian government filed a five-page document on 6 September 2011, stating that there were no less restrictive means available to achieve the purposes of the New South Wales and Queensland legislation other than detention in prison. The document (Australian Government, 2011) stated:

> Australia stresses that the community has a legitimate expectation to be protected from these offenders, and at the same time, that authorities owe these offenders a duty to try and [sic] rehabilitate them. The purpose of these schemes is not to indefinitely detain serious sex offenders, but rather to ensure as far as possible that their release into the community occurs in a way that is safe and respectful of the needs of both the community, and the offenders themselves.

Darren O'Donovan and Patrick Keyzer (2015) have described these communications and the Australian government's response as providing:

> a stark example of what may be termed normative dissension between an international body and a nation state, illustrating the dynamics of 'decoupling', where a state effectively separates its international legal commitments from practical implementation … [E]ven rich, developed, liberal democracies can pursue a policy of deliberate and persistent noncompliance. Ultimately, access to international justice in this context is

meaningless if the parties to international human rights instruments fail to comply.

(p. 148)

Anthony Lavender (2002) has referred to conflicting societal attitudes towards those considered dangerous as revolving around 'punishment', 'keeping society safe' and 'treatment and care' (p. S49). He points out that emphasising treatment and care may lead to perceptions of policymakers being 'too soft' on those considered dangerous, with calls for punishment and community safety being more important. As the title of this chapter indicates, there is an ongoing tension between the concepts of containment and rehabilitation. However, from a human rights perspective, the importance of the duty to rehabilitate offenders should be central to justifying breaching a person's liberty after a sentence has been served.

Containment alone offends against not only human rights, but well-established legal principles such as the principles of proportionality and finality in sentencing, the principle that governments should punish criminal conduct, not criminal types, and the principle against double punishment. There is thus good reason to consider rehabilitation together with containment rather than assume that one must exist without the other. That leads to a consideration of which management and treatment programs can facilitate rehabilitation.

Current mandated treatment options

Multiple existing programs aim to reduce reoffending. For example, in Victoria, therapeutic interventions are delivered by the Specialised Offender Assessment and Treatment Service and include both group and individual treatment and range from intensive to maintenance programs. While programs are delivered across both prison and community correctional services, group treatment is the option generally available in prison and is also given priority in the community (Victorian Ombudsman, 2015).

There is some data indicating positive outcomes following mandated treatment. In relation to sex offenders, Karl Hanson and colleagues' (2009) meta-analysis found that treated sex offenders had average sexual and overall recidivism rates of 10.9% and 31.8% respectively, compared to 19.2% and 48.3% for untreated offenders, based on an average follow-up period of 4.7 years. Similar results were found in a meta-analysis conducted some six years later (Schmucker & Lösel, 2015). A separate study by Brian Lovins and colleagues (2009) reported that sex offenders considered at high risk of reoffending who completed intensive residential treatment were more than two times less likely to reoffend than high-risk sex offenders who were not provided with intensive treatment.

One program involving a broader group of those considered at high risk of (re)offending that has received positive evaluation is the Problem Behaviour

Program, conducted by a multidisciplinary team at Forensicare (McCarthy, Ogloff, & McEwan, 2015). This program is a community-based service which 'provides assessment and treatment to individuals with high-risk problem behaviours, including harmful sexual behaviours, violence, threatening, stalking and fire-setting' (McCarthy et al., 2015, p. 5). Results from a study of those referred to the program between 2006 and 2011 indicated that the largest single problem behaviour exhibited was violence, accounting for almost half of all referrals (McCarthy et al., 2015). One in six individuals was referred with multiple problem behaviours (McCarthy et al., 2015). The treatment provided is largely based on cognitive behaviour therapy and focuses on criminogenic needs in order to stop the problem behaviour (McEwan, MacKenzie, & McCarthy, 2013). An evaluation of the program found that reoffending rates were significantly lower for those who had completed or remained in treatment (McCarthy et al., 2015).

Factors that can underpin treatment effectiveness include program delivery and the therapeutic relationship, the treatment environment, and how the individual responds to the program. Roger Przybylski (2015) summarised states that 'rather than following a one-size-fits-all approach, treatment is apt to be most effective when it is tailored to the risks, needs, and offense dynamics of individual sex offenders' (p. 4).

The dominant theory guiding many rehabilitation programs for offenders is the RNR model, which is based on the principles of risk, need and responsivity (Andrews & Bonta, 2010). There have been various critiques of this model, including that it constructs a universal model of offenders which fails to consider age, gender or cultural differences (Spivakovsky, 2013). Devon Polaschek (2011) points out that in practice programs adhering to this model vary widely, but that there is 'diversity and depth to these offerings: they are far from being one-size-fits-all' (p. 34).

As stated in the previous section, there are human rights concerns in relation to post-sentence detention and supervision. There are also human rights considerations that apply to mandated treatment programs. For example, offenders with mental or intellectual impairments may fall within the ambit of the United Nations *Convention on the Rights of Persons with Disabilities*. The Committee on the Rights of Persons with Disabilities (2014) has stated that in relation to offenders with disabilities 'Treatment is a social control sanction and should be replaced by formal criminal sanctions for offenders whose involvement in crime has been determined … [s]entencing a person to treatment is … incompatible with article 14 [the right to liberty]' (para. 34). The reasoning here appears to be that persons with disabilities should not be singled out for mandated treatment because of their disability. Whether this extends to mandated treatment for problem behaviours is another matter. The latter approach may be more easily justifiable from a human rights perspective than providing treatment based on the characteristics of the offender.

To avoid human rights concerns, voluntary treatment is undoubtedly preferable to mandated treatment. However, some research indicates that post-conviction mandated treatment may be as effective as voluntary treatment, at least in relation to reducing substance use and associated criminal behaviour (Bright & Martire, 2013; Schaub et al., 2010). Sarak Manchak and colleagues (2014) examined the effect of mandated mental health treatment (primarily through court diversion programs) on the therapeutic alliance and concluded that while mandated treatment relationships involve more therapist control, they remained 'predominantly affiliative'. This indicates that it is the quality of the therapeutic relationship that predicts treatment outcomes, rather than whether the relationship is entered into voluntarily.

Treatment, whether mandated or voluntary, may not be enough on its own to rehabilitate those who have been convicted of serious crimes. A coordinated response which addresses individual needs may in fact lead to better outcomes for community protection.

Coordinated responses

Given the complex needs of certain high-risk offenders, it seems that the most effective interventions can only be delivered through intensive case management and coordinated service delivery together with governance arrangements aimed at targeting criminogenic and therapeutic needs. The Problem Behaviour Program discussed in the previous section provides an example of one institution, Forensicare, coordinating treatment. Other arrangements coordinate services and therapeutic interventions across institutions. This section outlines multi-agency public protection arrangements in the United Kingdom and the Multiple and Complex Needs Initiative in Victoria as examples of coordinated responses to the management and treatment of those considered at high risk of offending.

Multi-agency public protection arrangements

In the United Kingdom, services for certain high-risk offenders may be coordinated via Multi-Agency Public Protection Arrangements (MAPPAs). These were set up in England and Wales in 2000 under sections 67 and 68 of the *Criminal Justice and Court Services Act 2000* (and consolidated under the *Criminal Justice Act 2003*) and adopted in Scotland by the *Management of Offenders etc. (Scotland) Act 2005* and in Northern Ireland by the *Criminal Justice (NI) Order 2008* (Logan, 2011; Thomson, 2011).

In England and Wales, the 'responsible authorities' of the MAPPA include the National Probation Service, HM Prison Service and the police forces of England and Wales. MAPPAs are coordinated by the Public Protection Unit within the National Offender Management Service. Multi-Agency Public Protection Panels manage the 'critical few' who pose a high or very high risk of serious harm. They often have a media profile, and their management plan will consist of collaboration between 'key agencies in the delivery of an agreed plan for the community management of the offender' (Wood & Kemshall, 2007, p. 2). There is a statutory duty on the various service providers, specifically health, housing, social services, education, social security and employment services, youth offending teams and electronic monitoring providers to cooperate with the directions given by Multi-Agency Public Protection Panels. Lindsay Thomson (2011, p. 169) summarises the four core functions of these Panels in Scotland as:

- identification of MAPPA offenders;
- sharing of relevant information
- assessment of risk of serious harm; and
- management of risk of serious harm.

Thomson (2011, p. 169) also points out that four features of good practice are:

- defensible decisions;
- rigorous risk assessment;
- delivery of risk management plans that match identified public protection needs; and
- evaluation of performance to improve delivery.

In Scotland, in addition to Multi-Agency Public Protection Panels, a Risk Management Team is a multidisciplinary team which helps develop and oversee the implementation of a risk management plan for an offender subject to an order for lifelong restriction. The Team is led by a Case Manager, who is the central point of contact (Risk Management Authority, 2007). Each year the Risk Management Team reviews the implementation of the plan and develops an updated plan for the following year. The revised plan is then submitted to the Risk Management Authority for approval.

While not necessarily statute-based, many jurisdictions in the United States have similar arrangements for those with mental health problems under forensic assertive community treatment programs. There are also multi-agency 'round tables' in Germany and 'safety house' partnerships in The Netherlands that show some evidence of effectiveness (Thomson, Goethals, & Nedopil, 2016).

Multiple and Complex Needs Panel

An Australian example of a multidisciplinary panel which was set up under legislation to manage the needs of those considered to be displaying problem behaviour was the Multiple and Complex Needs Panel, established in Victoria under the *Human Services (Complex Needs) Act 2003*. When the Multiple and Complex Needs Initiative legislation was first introduced into Parliament, emphasis was placed on the fact that the individuals who would be made subject to the scheme were 'sometimes dangerous' and that they presented 'significant levels of risk to the community, to staff and to themselves through challenging behaviours that include aggressive and assaultive behaviour, as well as self-harming, and risk taking' (Parliament of Victoria 2003). The introduction of this legislation can thus be viewed as having dual purposes – the control of problem behaviour as well as the coordination of care and treatment services.

The Panel consisted of a permanent part-time Chairperson and up to 12 members with expertise and experience in fields such as mental health, disability, housing and community services and alcohol and other drug dependency. Decisions were made by a Panel consisting of the Chairperson, two community Panel members and a nominee of the Secretary of the Victorian Department of Human Services. The Panel's responsibilities included determining if a particular individual was eligible for the scheme, authorising comprehensive assessments, determining, reviewing, varying and extending Care Plans and appointing a Care Plan Coordinator. In 2007, the Multiple and Complex Needs Initiative was evaluated positively (KPMG, 2007), with 50% of the individuals involved showing behavioural improvements, although whether these improvements were concerned with lowered levels of aggression and assault was not specified.

The Panel was disbanded in May 2009, but the *Human Services (Complex Needs) Act 2009* continued the initiative under the auspices of the Victorian Department of Human Services, Department of Health and the Department of Justice, rather than under an independent statutory body. There are now eight regional panels that consider all potential referrals for eligibility and which approve, monitor and review all care plans. Regional panels comprise senior program managers, regionally funded sector representatives and the Regional Coordinator. A Central Eligibility and Review Group confirms the individual's eligibility for the initiative and if the individual is eligible, a Care Plan Coordinator is appointed.

In the report on the five years of the Panel, it was pointed out that Care Plan Coordination was a key element to the overall success of the Initiative (Hamilton & Elford, 2009). Having an independent statutory panel in place to oversee Care Plans and the coordination of services can ensure that services communicate more effectively, but the key role of Care Plan Coordinators suggests that the success of such initiatives may depend upon strong leadership (Rosenbaum, 2002; Steadman, 1992).

Conclusion

How to respect the human dignity of high-risk offenders with complex needs is an ongoing challenge. There are human rights concerns in relation to both containment and mandated treatment for those offenders considered at high risk of reoffending. While mandating treatment for problem behaviours has its drawbacks in that it may result in resentful passivity rather than lessening the risk of reoffending, it is nevertheless more defensible than containment alone. There is also research indicating that mandated treatment is as effective as voluntary treatment in relation to rehabilitating those who have been convicted of crimes or who have been ordered into treatment through court diversion programs.

Although containment alone may seem to be the answer to concerns about community protection, it is costly both in a financial sense and from a human rights perspective. Rehabilitation should be an integral part of any containment regime. Polaschek (2011) points out that some governments understand this and 'recognise the need to respond to scientific research alongside public anxiety about crime' (p. 21).

Multi-agency coordination of services and treatment for those with complex needs has been evaluated positively, but there is a need for further research into its effectiveness. Nevertheless, because such coordination goes beyond treatment to addressing accommodation, psychosocial and other needs, it provides the best chance for reducing reoffending and enhancing the protection of the community.

References

Andrews, D. A., & Bonta, J. (2010). *The psychology of criminal conduct* (5th ed.). New Providence NJ: Matthew Bender & Co Inc.

Australian Government (2011). *Response of the Australian Government to the Views of the Committee in Communication No. 1635/2007 Tillman v Australia and Communication No. 1629/2007 Fardon v Australia.* Canberra: Attorney-General's Department.

Blackstone, W. (1772). *Commentaries on the laws of England, Book IV.* Philadelphia: R Bell.

Bright, D. A., & Martire, K. A. (2013). Does coerced treatment of substance-using offenders lead to improvements in substance use and recidivism? A Review of the treatment efficacy literature. *Australian Psychologist* 43(1), 69–81.

Committee on the Rights of Persons with Disabilities (2014). *Concluding observations on the initial report of Denmark.* UN Doc CRPD/C/DNK/CO/1 (30 October 2014).

Committee on the Rights of Persons with Disabilities (2015). *Guidelines on article 14 of the Convention on the Rights of Persons with Disabilities: The right to liberty and security of persons with disabilities.* Geneva: Office of the High Commissioner on Human Rights, United Nations. www.ohchr.org/EN/HRBodies/CRPD/Pages/ConventionRightsPersonsWithDisabilities.aspx

Complex Adult Victim Sex Offender Management Review Panel (2015). *Advice on the legislative and governance models under the Serious Sex Offenders (Detention and Supervision) Act 2009 (Vic).* Melbourne: Department of Justice (Victoria).

Davis, M. R., & Ogloff, J. R. P. (2008) Risk assessment and the dangerous offender. In K. Fritzon & P. Wilson (Eds). *Forensic and criminal psychology: An Australasian perspective.* North Ryde, NSW: McGraw Hill Australia.

Egan, C. (2011, 18 April). Marlon Noble 'victims' don't recall sex crimes. *The West Australian*, p. 3.

Gooding, P., McSherry, B., Arstein-Kerslake, A., & Andrews, L. (2017). Unfitness to stand trial and the indefinite detention of persons with cognitive disabilities in Australia: Human rights challenges and proposals for change. *University of Melbourne Law Review* 40, 816–866.

Hamilton, M. & Elford, K. (2009). *The report on the five years of the Multiple and Complex Needs Panel 2004–2009*. Melbourne: Multiple and Complex Needs Panel.

Hamilton, M. (2010). People with complex needs and the criminal justice system. *Current Issues in Criminal Justice* 22(2), 307–324.

Hanson, R. K., Bourgon, G., Helmus, L., & Hodgson, S. (2009). *A meta-analysis of the effectiveness of treatment for sexual offenders: Risk, need, and responsivity.* Ottawa: Public Safety Canada.

Keyzer, P., & McSherry, B. (2015). The preventive detention of sex offenders: Law and practice. *University of New South Wales Law Review* 38(2), 784–814.

KPMG (2007). *Department of Human Services Evaluation of Multiple and Complex Needs Initiative: Final Report*. Melbourne: KPMG.

Lavender, A. (2002). Developing services for people with dangerous and severe personality disorders. *Criminal Behaviour and Mental Health* 12, S46–S53.

Logan, C. (2011). Managing high-risk personality disordered offenders: Lessons learned to date. In B. McSherry & P. Keyzer (Eds.), *Dangerous people: Policy, prediction, and practice* (pp. 233–247). New York: Routledge.

Lovins, B., Lowenkamp, C. T., & Latessa, E. J. (2009). Applying the risk principle to sex offenders: Can treatment make some sex offenders worse? *The Prison Journal*, 89, 344–357.

Manchak, S. M., Skeem, J. L., & Rook, K. S. (2014). Care, control, or both? Characterizing major dimensions of the mandated treatment relationship. *Law and Human Behavior* 38(1), 47–57.

McCarthy, J., Ogloff, J., & McEwan, T. (2015). *Evaluation of the Problem Behaviour Program: A community based program for the assessment and treatment of problem behaviours*. Melbourne: Forensicare and Centre for Forensic Behavioural Science, Swinburne University of Technology.

McEwan, T., MacKenzie, R. D., & McCarthy, J. (2013). The Problem Behaviour Program: Threat assessment and management in a community forensic mental health context. In J. R. Meloy & J. Hoffman (Eds.), *International handbook of threat assessment* (pp. 360–374). Oxford: Oxford University Press.

McSherry, B. (2005). Indefinite and preventative detention legislation: From caution to an open door. *Criminal Law Journal* 29(2), 94–110.

McSherry, B. (2014). *Managing fear: The law and ethics of preventative detention and risk assessment*. New York: Routledge.

McSherry, B. (2017). Preventive justice, risk of harm and mental health law. In T. Tulich, R. Ananian-Walsh, S. Bronitt & S. Murray (Eds.), *Regulating preventive justice: Principle, policy and paradox* (pp. 61–74). London: Routledge.

McSherry, B., & Keyzer, P. (2009). *Sex offenders and preventive detention: Politics, policy and practice*. Sydney: Federation Press.

McSherry, B,. & Keyzer, P. (Eds.) (2011). *Dangerous people: Policy, prediction, and practice*. New York: Routledge.

O'Donovan, D., & Keyzer, P. (2015). 'Visions of a distant millennium'? The effectiveness of the UN human rights petition system. In P. Keyzer, V. Popovski & C. Sampfor (Eds.), *Access to international justice* (pp. 148–177). Oxford: Routledge.

Parliament of Victoria (2003). *Hansard: Legislative Assembly.* Human Services (Complex Needs) Bill, Second Reading, B. Pike, Minister for Health (27 August).

Polaschek, D. L. L. (2011). Many sizes fit all: A preliminary framework for conceptualizing the development and provision of cognitive-behavioral rehabilitation programs for offenders, *Aggression and Violent Behavior* 16, 20–35.

Przybylski, R. (2015). *Sex offender management assessment and planning initiative research brief: The effectiveness of treatment for adult sexual offenders.* Washington, DC: Office of Sex Offender Sentencing, Monitoring, Apprehending, Registering, and Tracking, U.S. Department of Justice.

Risk Management Authority (Scotland) (2007). *Risk Management Authority Standards and Guidelines: Risk management of offenders subject to an order for lifelong restriction.* Paisley: Risk Management Authority.

Rosenbaum, D. P. (2002). Evaluating multi-agency anti-crime partnerships: Theory, design, and measurement issues. *Crime Prevention Studies* 14, 171–225.

Schaub, M., Stevens, A., Berto, D., Hunt, N., Kerschl, V., McSweeney, T., Oeuvray, K., Puppo, I., Santa Maria, A., Trinkl, B., Werdenich, W., & Uchtenhagen, A. (2010). Comparing outcomes of 'voluntary' and 'quasi-compulsory' treatment of substance dependence in Europe. *European Addiction Research* 16(1), 53–60.

Schmucker, M., & Lösel, F. (2015). The effects of sexual offender treatment on recidivism: An international meta-analysis of sound quality evaluations, *Journal of Experimental Criminology* 11, 597–630.

Smith, C., & Nolan, M. (2016). Post-sentence continued detention of high-risk terrorist offenders in Australia. *Criminal Law Journal* 40, 163–179.

Spivakovsky, C. (2013). *Racialized correctional governance: The mutual constructions of race and criminal justice.* Farnham, UK: Ashgate.

Steadman, H. J. (1992). Boundary spanners: A key component for the effective interactions of the justice and mental health systems. *Law and Human Behavior* 16(1), 75–87.

Thomson, L. (2011). The role of forensic mental health services in managing high-risk offenders. In B. McSherry & P. Keyzer (Eds.), *Dangerous people: Policy, prediction, and practice* (pp. 165–181). New York: Routledge.

Thomson, L., Goethals, K., & Nedopil, N. (2016). Editorial – multi agency working in forensic psychiatry: theory and practice in Europe. *Criminal Behaviour and Mental Health* 26, 153–160.

Victorian Ombudsman (2015). *Investigation into the rehabilitation and reintegration of prisoners in Victoria.* Melbourne: Victorian Government Printer.

Wood, J., & Kemshall, H. (2007). *The operation and experience of Multi-Agency Public Protection Arrangements (MAPPA).* London: Home Office.

Young, M. B. (2015). *From commitment to culture: The 2015 Review of the Charter of Human Rights and Responsibilities Act 2006.* Melbourne: Victorian Government Printer.

Cases

Re Fardon v Australia [2010], Human Rights Committee, Communication No. 1629/
2007, UN Doc. CCPR/C/98/D/1629/2007 (12 April 2010).
Re Tillman v Australia [2010], Human Rights Committee, Communication No. 1635/
2007, UN Doc. CCPR/C/98/D/1635/2007 (12 April 2010).
Fardon v Attorney-General (Qld) [2004] 223 CLR 575.

Legislation

*Convention on the Rights of Persons with Disabilities: resolution adopted by the UN
General Assembly*, 24 January 2007. UN Doc: A/RES/61/106
Crimes (High Risk Offenders) Act 2006 (NSW)
Crimes (Serious Sex Offenders) Amendment Act 2013 (NSW)
Criminal Justice and Court Services Act 2000 (UK)
Criminal Justice (Northern Ireland) Order 2008 (NI)
Criminal Law Amendment Act 1945 (Qld)
Criminal Law (Sentencing) Act 1998 (SA)
Dangerous Prisoners (Sexual Offenders) Act 2003 (Qld)
Dangerous Sexual Offenders Act 2006 (WA)
International Covenant on Civil and Political Rights, 15 December 1966, UNTS vol.
999, p. 171.
Management of Offenders etc. (Scotland) Act 2005 (Scot.)
Penalties and Sentences Act 1992 (Qld)
Sentencing Act 1991 (Vic)
Sentencing Act 1995 (NT)
Sentencing Act 1995 (WA)
Sentencing Act 1997 (Tas)
Serious Sex Offenders Act 2013 (NT)
Serious Sex Offenders (Detention and Supervision) Act 2009 (Vic)

Chapter 13

Therapeutic jurisprudence and procedural justice in mental health practice

Responding to 'vulnerability' without coercion

Penelope Weller

Compulsory mental health treatment is a central feature of mental health systems throughout the developed world, despite the strong narrative of individual rights that dominated the mental health law debate in the second half of the 20th century (Weller, 2014). Rights-based mental health laws typically modify or balance legislative powers that permit compulsory mental health treatment with procedural protections (Weller, 2010). In conjunction with the dismantling of stand-alone mental health institutions across the developed world in the later decades of the 20th century, laws that permit compulsory mental health treatment were gradually extended to the community (see Chapter 2, this volume).

Compulsory mental health treatment is a form of protective paternalism invoked by the state to protect its citizens (Weller, 2017). The logic of benevolent paternalism is deeply embedded in the law's response to the vulnerable (Weller, 2017). Such laws have existed since Roman times, emerging formally in the 16th century as the *parens patriae* jurisdiction of the English courts, in which the state or sovereign stood in the role of protective father, and in the 17th century as the 'best interests' principle (Lush, 2014). *Parens patriae* and best interests applied to children, the elderly, the sick, the disabled and the mentally ill and all those in need of medical care (Then, 2013, p. 136). In the 21st century *parens patriae* remains the legal basis for interventions taken by the state to promote the health or social health of 'vulnerable' individuals (Weller, 2017).

Whereas vulnerable individuals were typically defined by their membership of a vulnerable group, the contemporary emphasis is on the practical decision-making ability or risk status of individuals (Weller, 2013a). In the mental health context, modern protective paternalism in the form of compulsory treatment is reserved for those who lack mental capacity (and are therefore unable to make rational decisions for themselves), those who are acutely unwell (and are therefore unable to make decisions) or those who are judged to be a serious risk to themselves or others (Weller, 2010). Such laws are justified on the basis that intervention on health grounds provides important and fundamental protections in a civilised society (Weller, 2011a).

Debates arising from the *Convention on the Rights of Persons with Disabilities* (CRPD), however, have challenged the validity of protective paternalism by crafting a radical reinterpretation of the principles of non-discrimination and equality before the law (Weller, 2013b). Rather than permitting a separate legal regime for those who lack mental capacity, as is currently the case, the CRPD insists that people with disabilities receive equal benefit and protection of the law (Lawson, 2008). In this model the recognition of different needs and abilities is envisaged as 'reasonable accommodation' of one's disability within the mainstream system (Mégret & Msipa, 2014). With respect to compulsory mental health treatment, the United Nations Committee on the Rights of People with Disabilities (CRPD) has indicated that such laws are no longer acceptable (2014, General Comment 1). The international human rights framework requires the abolition of compulsory mental health treatment (Arstein-Kerslake & Flynn, 2016). In developed nations the CRPD has amplified the debate about the clinical, ethical and legal status of compulsory treatment orders, but has not yet resulted in substantive legal change consistent with international human rights principles.

This chapter looks beyond the traditional emphasis on protection to explore the connections between therapeutic jurisprudence and arguments against compulsion put forward by consumers and survivors of mental health services. The aim is to provide an alternative vision of a mental health system based on voluntary (rather than compulsory) treatment. The key argument is that therapeutic justice (TJ)/procedural justice (PJ) complements the human rights approach and recovery-oriented practice in mental health and provides a method that can mobilise systemic and legal change away from compulsory treatment. The first part of the chapter explores the emerging literature on the effects of coercion in mental health care. The second part explores the concept of TJ, arguing that the key contribution of TJ to mental health is its emphasis on the role of decision-makers, in the case of mental health psychiatrists and tribunals, as active legal agents. The third part of the chapter discusses the potential contribution of PJ, showing how PJ literature illustrates the overarching social and behavioural benefits that flow from just and fair practice.

The critique of coercion

The critique of compulsory treatment by the consumer movement dates from the earliest consumer literature (Chamberlin, 1978; Szasz, 2007). Considered as a whole, the literature can be grouped into three main themes. One theme relates to the limited health benefits of compulsory treatment in light of the burdensome side effects of psychotropic medication; another relates to the correlation between poor-quality care and compulsion; and a third relates to the experience of compulsory treatment itself.

The argument that compulsory treatment fails to provide the benefit it claims is adopted by an active international alliance between psychiatrists, psychologists, survivors of psychiatry and human right activists (Kallert, Mezzich & Monahan, 2011). The key point in this literature is that grave intrusion upon individual liberty occasioned by compulsory mental health treatment should be clearly justified in terms of health benefits and positive social outcomes. The effort to develop an evidence base for compulsion, however, has foundered. As is noted in Chapter 1 of this collection it is now well recognised that the scientific evidence in support of compulsory treatment is ambivalent at best. Three large international randomised controlled trials, the 'gold standard' in clinical research, have failed to identify significant improvements in health or social outcomes amongst those who are subject to compulsory treatment (Burns et al., 2013; Churchill et al., 2007; Rugkåsa & Dawson, 2013; Rugkåsa, Dawson & Burns, 2014; Steadman et al., 2001; Swartz, 1999).

On the other hand, the association between compulsory treatment and poor care continues to be documented. A volume of essays on coercion in psychiatry (2011) notes confusion around the concept of coercion coupled with a dearth of literature and research exploring the impact of coercion on therapeutic relationships (Kallert et al., 2011). A second volume (2013) similarly notes that the role of coercion in mental health care is under-theorised and poorly understood (Dennis & Monahan, 2013, p. 18). Hiday, Diamond and Lopez observe strong correlations between the use of coercion and poor quality of services (Dennis & Monahan, 2013, pp. 3–4). Similarly, Manuel et al. (2013) found that the increased use of coercive strategies was associated with stigmatising beliefs about the mentally ill. An Australian volume entitled *Coercive care* also explores these issues (Freckelton & McSherry, 2013). Some authors have urged a deeper engagement with the experience of consumers as an avenue for future research (Oaks, 2011; Russo & Wallcraft, 2011).

In this vein, Australian researcher Edwina Light and her colleagues find that the experience of coercion in mental illness is associated with a high degree of distress. They observe that the experience of mental illness is 'characterised by intense practical, moral, existential and legal complexity and uncertainty' (Light et al., 2014). Their research shows that distress emerges not only from the mental illness itself, but from the sense of isolation and disempowerment that arises from the experience of being subject to compulsion, from communication gaps, and from the difficulty in obtaining optimal care and accessing mental health services. Light et al. describe the use of compulsory treatment as central to consumer accounts of vulnerability, trauma, isolation and agency. They argue the experience reflects a 'kind of deprivation or social injustice faced by many sufferers from severe mental illness' (2014, p. 348) that was as much about treatment and care and coercion as it was about the person's individual situation. Reflecting on the logic of paternalism, Light points to the 'uneasy elision between the duty of care for patients and the responsibility to act for society' (Thornicroft & Henderson, 2016, p. 647).

Consumer advocate Mary O'Hagan also identifies compulsory treatment as a violent contradiction at the heart of mental health policy. She argues that recovery-oriented practice, which has become a centrepiece of mental health policy and practice models in many English-speaking countries, is undermined by compulsory mental health treatment.

> The four cornerstones of a recovery approach are hope and belief in people's potential, self-determination over their lives, the choice of a broad range of services, and equal participation in their communities ... Legal coercion erodes all the cornerstones of the recovery philosophy, yet it remains a core response in our mental health systems.
>
> (O'Hagan, 2012)

O'Hagan reminds us of the real and immediate consequences of compulsory treatment. This includes the experience of being apprehended by mental health professionals and police, forcibly injected, detained in hospital (and sometimes in seclusion) and compelled to take treatment. Compulsory treatment is itself a significant traumatic event.

Despite the lack of evidence in support of compulsion and the mounting evidence against it, attempts to displace compulsory treatment practices have proved difficult. Recent studies of innovative practice in mental health show that approaches designed to reduce compulsory treatment and coercion in psychiatry, such as recovery-oriented practice and advance directives, are actively resisted by psychiatrists and/or poorly implemented by mental health staff (Thornicroft & Henderson, 2016). The logic of compulsion and the belief that compulsive treatment is efficacious, it seems, is entrenched in the mental health sector.

In a recent review of published research studies, de Jong et al. (2016) report that advance statements reduce the occurrence of compulsory admissions (and hence compulsory treatment) by approximately one-quarter when compared with other measures such as medication compliance enhancement, integrated treatment and compulsory treatment orders. The term 'advance statements' is used by De Jong et al. as an umbrella term for a range of decision-making interventions that vary with respect to their basis in legislation and the manner in which health professionals are involved in their creation. De Jong et al.'s review indicates that forms of advance statements that incorporate a joint crisis plan and are predicated on the empowerment of consumers are likely to achieve the best clinical results. Why this might be so, or how the benefits of empowerment might be harnessed in the clinical enterprise is yet to be fully explored in the mental health context. As is explored in the next section, current research in TJ and PJ helps shed light on these issues.

Therapeutic jurisprudence

Therapeutic jurisprudence (TJ) is a portable legal theory or philosophy and a field of empirical study that recognises law as 'therapeutic agent' (Wexler, 1999). TJ sees the law as a social force that may have therapeutic or anti-therapeutic consequences. It concentrates on the impact of the law (which includes rules of law, legal procedures and roles of legal actors) on emotional life and on 'individual wellbeing' (King, 2008a, p. 1097). This approach is sometimes referred to as 'emotionally intelligent justice' (Winick, 1997, p. 185a). In Australia, TJ perspectives have influenced the establishment of problem-solving courts that are characterised by active judging and 'wrap around' services (Wexler, 2014). Problem-solving courts are structured to invite active listening and displays of empathy, all aimed at soliciting active participation by the parties and encouraging solution-focused judging (King 2009). Respectful treatment and the opportunity for self-determination are also important components of the approach (King, 2008b).

Therapeutic jurisprudence theorists assert that '(t)he underlying philosophy of solution-focused judging therapeutic jurisprudence can be applied in judging in any context' (King, 2009, p. 184). In the mental health context, solution-focused judging has influenced the practice of mental health review tribunals, but has not been applied to the clinical context, although there are clear parallels with some models of recovery-oriented practice (Weller, 2011b). For example, in Victoria the Mental Health Tribunal is explicitly encouraged to adopt a solution-focused approach.

Therapeutic jurisprudence augments recovery-oriented practice by facilitating the recognition of the way coercive legal powers impact on the clinical context. It allows us to see that clinical decision-makers are legal actors, with legal powers, whose actions with respect to the administration of the law may support (or undermine) individual well-being (Wexler, 1999). Compulsory treatment powers bring the law into the clinical context. If clinical staff, who are charged with the implementation of the law, were to actively consider their role as legal actors, they might consider using a TJ approach to implement their legal mandate. Understanding that the law, in this case in the form of compulsory treatment powers, has emotional and psychological impacts on the well-being of individuals opens the way for a TJ approach.

Therapeutic jurisprudence encourages an explicit engagement with the law as a therapeutic (or non-therapeutic) agent (Brookbanks, 2015, p. 5). It invites legal actors, in this case clinical staff, to consider their actions and to recognise the impact of the law. TJ is said to 'reach out to explore models of practice that are more relationally engaged, less adversarial, more psychologically beneficial and more capable of producing non-exploitative outcomes'

(Wexler, 2014, p. 6). In the context of mental health, TJ perspectives enable staff to consider the broader impact of their role, beyond a limited view of clinical expertise. It asks them to accept responsibility for the impacts and effects of the system, to recognise the impact of the law and adopt practices that may ameliorate its negative effects.

Procedural justice

The key to the development of appropriate therapeutic practice with respect to coercion lies in the body of literature referred to as procedural justice (PJ). In the mental health context, PJ provides a helpful basis for understanding the role that coercion – or its absence – plays in the provision of mental health treatment.

Procedural justice scholarship developed from research on the psychology of justice that began to trace subjective perceptions of the fairness of a decision-making procedure in the mid-1970s (Thibaut & Walker, 1975). PJ scholarship is broadly concerned with the question of why people obey the law, but is specifically focused on understanding why people are more willing to accept court decisions if they believe court procedures are fair (see Casper, Tyler & Fisher, 1988; Lind et al., 1993; Maccoun et al., 1988; Tyler & Huo, 2002). The PJ research shows that, regardless of the outcome, satisfaction is increased when people believe that all parties have the opportunity to present their case; that the decision-makers have received the necessary information; and when they believe that the decision-makers will consider the information or evidence impartially and apply to rules consistently across a number of cases (Meares & Tyler, 2014; see also Galligan, 1996; Solum, 2004). The research shows that decisions are respected and followed because people value fair decision-making process more than the outcomes of decisions (Moorhead, Sefton & Scanlan, 2008). People's responses are closely associated with trust and legitimacy. Legal actors must be 'fair' and must be 'seen as being fair' (Meares & Tyler, 2014). Fairness involves transparency in procedures, explanation of rules and decisions, and the promotion of procedures that give interested parties a voice in the proceedings. This formulation sounds very similar to the Australian concept of natural justice/procedural fairness. PJ, however, emphasises the subjective perception of fairness held by participants in the legal process and its psychological effects.

Procedural justice research shows when the conditions of fairness are met, positive behaviours are elicited and sustained over time. For example, Dillon and Emery (1996) found that nine years after a custody hearing, those parents who thought the hearing was procedurally fair had 'more frequent current contact with their children and greater involvement in current decisions about them' (p. 131; see also Tyler et al., 2007). The PJ research therefore challenges the idea the people are interested in fairness for instrumental or self-interested reasons. Rather, the research shows that people are concerned with a broader set of issues about fairness that relate to the perceived relationship between figures of authority and members of different social groups (Meares & Tyler, 2014; see also Tyler & Lind, 1992). This is described as the relational component of justice. The way people:

> are treated by legal authorities provides them with information about how that authority views them and the group or groups to which they belong. In other words, the way people interpret the fairness of procedures has a substantial relational component.
>
> (Meares & Tyler, 2014, p. 527)

The PJ literature suggests that people value the relational component of procedural justice because it conveys a feeling of dignity and respect and a message of inclusion. PJ scholars argue that respect for a person's rights indicates respect for the rights of the person's social group. If people are treated as marginal, or treated differently than others, they feel devalued, socially inferior and undesirable. But when people who are members of a group, organisation, community or society deal with an authority and 'see evidence that fair procedures are shaping decisions, rules, and policies, then they merge their sense of self with the group, intertwining their identities with group values' (Meares & Tyler, 2014, p. 538). In effect, people who identify with institutions and authorities accept decisions and cooperate with authorities because to do so contributes to the standing of their group (Tyler, 2011; Tyler & Blader, 2000). People trust institutions and accept authority when institutions demonstrate respect and trustworthiness to the group (Welsh, Stienstra & McAdoo, 2013). Fairness is also relational in the broader sense of the law itself being just.

Amy Ronner summarises the PJ principles as voice, neutrality, validation, respect and voluntariness (Tyler, 2006a). Voice refers to the opportunity to explain one's concerns; neutrality refers to evidence or belief that decisions are being made on facts and without partiality; respect refers to the treatment of people with respect, courtesy and dignity, which in turn elicit the dimension of trustworthiness (King, 2008a); and voluntariness refers to the principle that participation in the law must always be freely chosen by the person as a matter of choice (Ronner, 2002; see also Tyler, 2006a). Tyler and colleagues similarly identify the four fundamental elements of PJ as neutrality, participation, dignity and trustworthiness (Tyler & Blader, 2003; Tyler & Bies, 1990). Tyler and Blader (2003) also describe a four-part model of PJ that encompasses the adoption of practices of fairness and response by decision-makers such as impartiality, good faith and taking an 'outsiders' or fresh view of offender's behaviour, generating a personal or subjective sense of dignity and fairness in those who participate in the justice system. In demonstrating that people see respect for these values as more important that the outcome of decisions, PJ confirms an important observation – that how we do things trumps what we do.

Application of procedural justice

How does PJ help in the clinical context? PJ research shows that individual acceptance of authority, whether that be the authority of psychiatrists or the authority of the tribunal, is more likely when the person is treated with dignity and respect. For example, Paternoster et al. (1997) found that people are more likely to follow a decision based on an internal commitment to it.

The PJ literature also shows that when respectful actions are the norm, that is, when individuals see that respect and dignity are accorded to the group to which they belong, the likelihood that the person will cooperate with authoritative direction is also increased. For example, Tyler and colleagues found that people were more likely to accept and follow the directions of legal authorities when they felt that the authorities' processes were fair and their motives legitimate (Tyler, 1996; 2006a; Tyler & Huo, 2002). Writing in the context of offenders with mental health issues, Kopelovich et al. (2013) observed that when they were treated with respect, offenders' perceptions of procedural justice improved over time and were positively associated with offenders' hope in their recovery and with reduced symptoms. The authors argue that people with severe mental illness and members of other stigmatised groups may be particularly responsive to procedural justice (Kopelovich et al., 2013).

On the other hand, it is observed that the failure to accord respect elicits resistance and noncompliance. For example, Bruce Winick (1992) argues coercion and paternalism in legal processes are likely to promote non-compliance. In describing the negative effects of coercive policing on one hand, and the positive effect of fairness and procedural justice on the other, Tom Tyler concludes that the use of coercion or force by individuals in authority and the associated failure to respect or acknowledge the dignity of the person increases resistance and non-compliance (Tyler, 2006a; 2011). Elsewhere, Winick has argued that being labelled 'incompetent', even where procedural safeguards exist to challenge such a determination, induces feelings of helplessness and impedes the basic human need for self-determination and self-actualisation. This leads to non-participation in decisions that are central to living a full life (Winick, 1995). Applied to psychiatric settings, these observations suggest that patterns of coercion and resistance are created by certain styles of interpersonal interaction (Tyler, 1996). It is likely that dynamics of this type also occur in health and mental health care settings. Tyler's point is that people strive toward self-management, and are encouraged to do so when offered respect and dignity from a legitimate authority, but they will also seek to disrupt authority if respect is not forthcoming or the authority is seen as illegitimate (Tyler, 2006b; Tyler & Bies, 1990; Tyler & Huo, 2002).

The concept of legitimacy is given a broad meaning. The PJ literature shows that cooperation is increased when people perceive the process of the institution to be fair and to be fairly applied to everyone. Fairness in this sense refers not only to the fair application of the law, but to the recognition that the law itself is just and fair. In other words, PJ speaks to the substance of the law. It points to the importance of fairness and equity as principles underlying the rule of law. A fundamental problem with coercive treatment in mental health is that mental health law provides a legal framework for people with mental illness that differs from that applied to people with other health problems. In this sense, it fails a fundamental test. Prior to the CRPD, rights-based approaches to mental health law reform accepted the proposition that it is appropriate to place those who lack mental capacity because of mental illness under the care of a psychiatrist, provided legal oversight was provided (Weller, 2010). It is this distinction that is challenged by the CRPD (Arstein-Kerslake & Flynn, 2016). The PJ literature suggests that fairness, transparency and the adoption of an actively respectful and open stance by clinicians and others will invoke active cooperation with the clinical enterprise. This conclusion contrasts with the idea that the imposition of treatment 'for one's own good' is appropriate. This is because such actions privilege a clinical assessment of what is the best outcome. It reorients the notion of 'best outcome' toward a holistic consideration of an individual's life.

The PJ research shows that the relational outcomes (not the clinical outcomes) are likely to be the most valued, and more likely to be associated with positive behaviours that are sustained over time. As Edwina Light's research suggests, the violation of dignity that is associated with compulsory treatment adds to the profound sense of confusion and disintegration that is reported by those who suffer from mental illness. TJ/PJ literature indicates that coercive powers are likely to have a negative impact. In summary, a TJ/PJ approach to the mental health context facilitates a whole-of-system approach, counters the clinical discourse that currently dominates mental health research, inserts interdisciplinary insights into the compulsory treatment debate, and encourages health professionals to fully recognise and acknowledge their role as legal actors. In short, the TJ/PJ literature points to the notion of respect as a method or approach by which voluntary treatment can be achieved.

Conclusion

This chapter has considered the questions raised by the observation that compulsory mental health treatment can no longer be considered acceptable. On one hand, many people who provide care in health and social settings witness terrible human suffering and wish to respond to it. On the other, those who are subject to such intervention by the state point to the weight of negative personal experiences with intrusive coercive practices. Some consumers of mental health services who have been subject to compulsory intervention point to underlying social and scientific discourses that pathologise and marginalise social difference (Shakespeare, 2013, p. 93). If compulsory mental health treatment is disallowed, what institutional mechanism can be put in its place?

The TJ/PJ literature intervenes in the debate about compulsory treatment in mental health by observing that treating people with respect has immediate and long-term clinical, social and political benefits. In the mental health context, the literature points to the conclusion that TJ/PJ theory and practice will be useful because it allows the connections between dignity, autonomy, freedom, choice, the human rights framework and recovery to become visible. Such an approach is compatible with the human rights framework the CRPD requires.

Therapeutic jurisprudence/procedural justice perspectives complement both the human rights approach and recovery-oriented practice in mental health by providing a method that can mobilise systemic and legal change. When compulsory treatment powers are part of the law, PJ practice provides a method for ameliorating its worst effects. The research shows that the maximum benefits of PJ will only be achieved if the law itself is perceived as fair. On this basis, PJ provides a robust evidence base to support the abolition of statutorily mandated compulsory medical treatment, and its replacement with a fair and equitable legal framework.

References

Arstein-Kerslake, A., & Flynn, E. (2016). The General Comment on Article 12 of the Convention on the Rights of Persons with Disabilities: A roadmap for equality before the law. *The International Journal of Human Rights* 20, 471–490.

Brookbanks, W. J. (2015). *Therapeutic jurisprudence: New Zealand perspectives.* Wellington: Thomson Reuters.

Burns, T., Rugkåsa, J., Molodynski, A., Dawson, J., Yeeles, K., Vazquez-Montes, M., Voysey, M., Sinclair, J., & PriebeS. (2013). Community treatment orders for patients with psychosis: a randomised controlled trial (OCTET). *The Lancet* 381, 1627–1633.

Casper, D., Tyler, T., & Fisher, B. (1988). Procedural justice in felony cases. *Law and Society Review* 22(3), 483–508.

Chamberlin, J. (1978). *On our own: Patient-controlled alternatives to the mental health system.* New York: McGraw-Hill.

Churchill, R., Owen, G., Singh, S., & Hotopf, M. (2007). *International experiences of using community treatment orders.* London: Institute of Psychiatry.

Committee on the Rights of Persons with Disabilities (2014). *General Comment No 1 (2014), Article 12 Equal Recognition Before The Law,* 11th sess, UN Doc CRPD/C/GC/1 (19 May 2012).

Convention on the Rights of Persons with Disabilities, opened for signature 13 December 2006, 46 ILM 433 (entered into force 3 May 2008).

Dennis, D. L., & Monahan, J. (2013). *Coercion and aggressive community treatment: A new frontier in mental health law.* New York, NY: Springer Science & Business Media.

de Jong, M. H., Kamperman, A. M., Oorschot, M., Priebe, S., Bramer, W., van de Sande, R., Van Gool, A. R., & Mulder, C. L. (2016). Interventions to reduce compulsory psychiatric admissions: A systematic review and meta-analysis. *JAMA Psychiatry* 73(7), 657–664.

Dillon, P., & Emery, R., (1996). Divorce mediation and resolution of child custody disputes: Long-term effects. *American Journal of Orthopsychiatry* 66, 131–140.

Freckelton, I., & McSherry, B. (Eds.) (2013). *Coercive care*. London: Routledge.

Galligan, D.J. (1996). *Due process and fair procedures: A study of administrative procedures*. New York: Oxford University Press.

Kallert,. T., Mezzich, J., & Monahan, M. (Eds.) (2011). *Coercive treatment in psychiatry*. Oxford: Wiley-Blackwell.

King, M. (2008a). Restorative justice, therapeutic jurisprudence and the rise of emotionally intelligent justice. *Melbourne University Law Review* 32, 1096–1126.

King, M. (2008b). Problem-solving court judging, therapeutic jurisprudence and transformational leadership. *Journal of Judicial Administration* 17, 155–177.

King, M. S. (2009). *Solution focused judging bench book*. Melbourne: Australian Institute of Judicial Administration.

Kopelovich, S., Yanos, P., Pratt, C., & Koernerc, J. (2013). Procedural justice in mental health courts: Judicial practices, participant perceptions, and outcomes related to mental health recovery. *International Journal of Law and Psychiatry* 36, 113–120.

Lawson, A. (2008). People with psychosocial impairments or conditions, reasonable accommodation and the Convention on the Rights of Persons with Disabilities. *Law in Context* 26(2), 62–84.

Light, E. M., Robertson, M. D., Boyce, P., Carney, T., Rosen, A., Cleary, M., Hunt, G. E., O'Connor, N., Ryan, C., & Kerridge, I. H. (2014). The lived experience of involuntary community treatment: A qualitative study of mental health consumers and carers. *Australasian Psychiatry* 22(4), 345–351.

Lind, E. A., Kulik, C. T., Ambrose, M., & de Vera Park, M. V. (1993). Individual and corporate dispute resolution: Using procedural fairness as a decision heuristic. *Administrative Science Quarterly* 38, 224–251.

Lush, D. (2014). Roman origins of modern guardianship law. In K. Dayton, (Ed.), *Comparative perspectives on adult guardianship* (pp. 3–15). Durham, North Carolina: Carolina Academic Press.

Maccoun, R., Lind, E., Hensler, D., Bryant, D., & Ebener, P. (1988). *Alternative adjudication: An evaluation of the New Jersey automobile program*. Santa Monica, CA: The Institute for Civil Justice.

Manuel, J., Appelbaum, P. S., Le Melle, S. M., Mancini, A. D., Huz, S., Stellato, C. B., & Finnerty, M. T. (2013). Use of intervention strategies by assertive community treatment teams to promote patient engagement. *Psychiatric Services* 64(6), 579–585.

Meares, T. L., & Tyler, T. R. (2014). Justice Sotomayor and the jurisprudence of procedural justice. *The Yale Law Journal Forum* [online], 525–549.

Mégret, F., & Msipa, D. (2014). Global reasonable accommodation: How the Convention on the Rights of Persons with Disabilities changes the way we think about equality. *South African Journal on Human Rights* 30(2), 252–274.

Moorhead, R., Sefton, M., & Scanlan, L. (2008). *Just satisfaction?: What drives public and participant satisfaction with courts and tribunals*. London: Ministry of Justice.

Oaks, D. W. (2011). The moral imperative for dialogue with organizations of survivors of coerced psychiatric human rights violations. In T.W. Kallert, J. E. Mezzich & J. Monahan (Eds.), *Coercive treatment in psychiatry: Clinical, legal and ethical aspects* (pp. 187–212). Chichester, West Sussex: John Wiley & Sons.

O'Hagan, M. (2012). Legal coercion: The elephant in the recovery room. www.scot tishrecovery.net/resource/legal-coercion-the-elephant-in-the-recovery-room/

Paternoster, R.Bachman, R., Brame, R., & Sherman, L. W. (1997). Do fair procedures matter? The effect of procedural justice on spouse assault. *Law & Society Review* 31, 163–204.

Ronner, A. (2002). Songs of validation, voice and voluntary participation: Therapeutic jurisprudence, Miranda and juveniles. *University of Cincinnati Law Review* 71, 89–114.

Rugkåsa, J., & Dawson, J. (2013). Community treatment orders: Current evidence and the implications. *The British Journal of Psychiatry* 203(6), 406–408.

Rugkåsa, J., Dawson, J., & Burns, T. (2014). CTOs: What is the state of the evidence? *Social Psychiatry & Psychiatric Epidemiology* 49(12), 1861–1871.

Russo, J., & Wallcraft, J. (2011). Resisting variables – service user/survivor perspectives on researching coercion. In *Coercive treatment in psychiatry: Clinical, legal and ethical aspects* (pp. 213–234). Chichester, West Sussex: John Wiley & Sons.

Shakespeare, T. (2013). Nasty, brutish, and short? On the predicament of disability and embodiment. In J. E. Bickenbach, F. Felder and B. Schmitz (Eds.), *Disability and the good human life*. Cambridge: Cambridge University Press.

Solum, L. B. (2004). Procedural justice. *Southern California Law Review* 78, 183–190.

Steadman, H. J., Gounis, K., Dennis, D., Hopper, K., Roche, B., Swartz, M., & Robbins, P. C. (2001). Assessing the New York City involuntary outpatient commitment pilot program. *Psychiatric Services* 52, 330–336

Swartz, M. S., (1999). Can involuntary outpatient commitment reduce hospital recidivism?: Findings from a randomized trial with severely mentally ill individuals. *American Journal of Psychiatry* 156, 1968–1975

Szasz, T. (2007). *Coercion as cure: A critical history of psychiatry*. New Brunswick, NJ: Edison Transaction Publishers.

Then, S. N.- (2013). *Evolution* and innovation in guardianship laws: Assisted decision-making. *Sydney Law Review* 35, 133–166.

Thibaut, J., & Walker, L. (1975). *Procedural justice: A psychological analysis*. Hillsdale, New Jersey: Lawrence Erlbaum.

Thornicroft, G., & Henderson, C. (2016). Editorial: Joint decision making and reduced need for compulsory psychiatric admission. *JAMA Psychiatry* 73(7), 647–648.

Tyler, T. R. (1996). The psychological consequences of judicial procedures: Implications for civil commitment hearings. In D. B. Wexler & B. J. Winick (Eds.), *Law in a therapeutic key: Developments in therapeutic jurisprudence* (pp. 3–15). Durham, NC: Carolina Academic Press.

Tyler, T. R. (2006a). *Why people obey the law*. Princeton: Princeton University Press.

Tyler, T. R. (2006b). Legitimacy and legitimation. *Annual Review of Psychology* 57, 375–400.

Tyler, T. R. (2011). *Why people cooperate: The role of social motivations*. Princeton, New Jersey: Princeton University Press.

Tyler, T. R., & Bies, R., (1990). Beyond formal procedures: The interpersonal context of procedural justice. In J. Carroll (Ed.), *Applied social psychology and organizational settings* (pp. 77–98). Hillsdale, NJ: Erlbaum.

Tyler, T. R., & Blader, S. L. (2000). *Cooperation in groups: Procedural justice, social identity and behavioural engagement*. Philadelphia, PA: Psychology Press.

Tyler, T. R., & Blader, S. L. (2003). The group engagement model: Procedural justice, social identity, and cooperative behavior. *Personality and Social Psychology Review* 7(4), 349–361.

Tyler, T. R., & Huo, Y. J. (2002). *Trust in the law: Encouraging public cooperation with the police and courts*. New York: Russell Sage Foundation.

Tyler, T. R., & Lind, E. A. (1992). A relational model of authority in groups. *Advances in Experimental Social Psychology* 25, 115–191.

Tyler, T. R., Sherman, L., Strang, H., Barnes, G. C., Woods, D. (2007). Reintegrative shaming, procedural justice, and recidivism: The engagement of offenders' psychological mechanisms in the Canberra RISE drinking-and-driving experiment. *Law and Society Review* 41, 553–586.

Weller, P. (2010). Lost in translation: human rights and mental health law. In B. McSherry & P. Weller (Eds), *Rethinking rights–based mental health laws* (pp. 51–72). Oxford and Portland: Hart Publishing.

Weller, P. (2011a). The Convention on the Rights of Persons with Disabilities and the social model of health: New perspectives. *Journal of Mental Health Law* 21, 74–83.

Weller, P. (2011b). Taking a reflexive turn: Non-adversarial justice and mental health review tribunals. *Monash University Law Review* 37(1), 81–101.

Weller, P. (2013a). Towards a genealogy of coercive care. In I. Freckelton & B. McSherry (Eds.), *Coercive care* (pp. 15–30). London: Routledge.

Weller, P. (2013b). *New law and ethics in mental health advance directives: The Convention on the Rights of Person with Disabilities and the Right to Choose*. East Sussex: Routledge.

Weller, P. (2014). Governmentality and the CRPD: A radical critique of disability in law. *Griffith Law Review* 23(1), 498–518.

Weller, P. (2017). Substituted decision making. In A. M. Farrell, J. Devereux, I. Karpin & P. Weller (Eds.) *Health law: Frameworks and context* (pp. 127–137). Cambridge: Cambridge University Press.

Welsh, N., Stienstra, D., & McAdoo, B. (2013). The application of procedural justice research to judicial actions and techniques in settlement sessions. In T. Sourdin & A. Zariski (Eds.), *The multi-tasking judge: Comparative judicial dispute resolution* (pp. 57–86). Pyrmont, NSW: Thomson Reuters.

Wexler, D. (1999). Therapeutic jurisprudence: An overview. www.law.arizona.edu/dep ts/upr-intj/

Wexler, D. (2014). Moving forward on mainstreaming therapeutic jurisprudence: An ongoing process to facilitate the therapeutic design and application of the law. *Therapeutic Jurisprudence*, Paper 6.

Winick, B. J. (1992). On autonomy: Legal and psychological perspectives. *Villanova Law Review*, 37, 1705, 1715–1721.

Winick, B. J. (1995). The side effects of incompetency labelling and the implications for mental health. *Psychology, Public Policy, and Law* 1, 6–42.

Winick, B. J. (1997). The jurisprudence of therapeutic jurisprudence. *Psychology, Public Policy, and Law* 3(1), 184–206.

Chapter 14

Adult guardianship and its alternatives in Australia

John Chesterman

Guardianship

Guardianship is one of the principal means by which the decision-making authority of an adult can be legally removed. A guardianship order enables another person to substitute their decisions for those of the represented person. Other substitute decision-making processes include compulsory mental health treatment (e.g., under the *Mental Health Act 2014* Vic), activation of enduring powers of attorney (e.g., under the *Powers of Attorney Act 2014* Vic), and the making of medical treatment decisions by the highest-ranked person in a statutory hierarchy (e.g., under Part 4A of the *Guardianship and Administration Act 1986* Vic).

Australia's current guardianship laws were developed during the 1980s and were considered international leaders for their use of inquisitorial tribunal processes and for the creation of last-resort public guardians, beginning with the Office of the Public Advocate in Victoria in 1986 (Carney & Tait, 1997). In the decades since, all jurisdictions in Australia have developed their own guardianship laws and practices, with the Northern Territory being the last jurisdiction (in 2016) to adopt what might be termed modern guardianship laws with the establishment of a tribunal process for the making of guardianship orders, and the creation of an independent guardian of last resort (*Guardianship of Adults Act 2016* NT).

In Australia guardianship orders tend to be able to be made (e.g., *Guardianship and Administration Act 1986* Vic, sections 22, 46) if a person has 'a disability' which renders them unable 'to make reasonable judgements' and where that person 'is in need of' a guardian or administrator. Guardianship orders are made by tribunals. In Victoria, the guardianship list at the Victorian Civil and Administrative Tribunal (VCAT, 2015) shows that over 3,000 applications are made each year for guardianship and administration orders.

The Office of the Public Advocate (OPA) is Victoria's adult guardian of last resort. It is appointed as guardian on over 800 occasions each year (OPA, 2016). In 2015–16, OPA was appointed as guardian on 862 occasions, with a further 783 matters carried over from the previous year. Typically, more than one-third of OPA's guardianship clients have dementia. In 2015–16, 41% of OPA's guardianship clients had dementia, with mental ill health (31%), intellectual disability (29%) and acquired brain injuries (23%) constituting the next highest disability categories (a significant number of clients have more than one disability).

The term 'guardianship' can apply both to the appointment of a financial manager (known in Victoria as an administrator) and the appointment of a guardian, who, depending on the terms of the order, can make certain lifestyle decisions. In Victoria, the most common lifestyle decisions made when OPA is the guardian are accommodation decisions, followed by medical treatment decisions and then service provision decisions (OPA, 2015).

Guardianship is normally defined as a 'protective' measure rather than a coercive intervention. Guardians make decisions on behalf of the guardianship client, known as a 'represented person'. Usually represented persons do not actively object to the lifestyle decisions guardians make, such as determining where a person will live. When a represented person does actively object, for instance by regularly leaving the accommodation setting to which they have been moved, then the guardianship order will likely be considered unenforceable.

Guardianship decisions are, however, coercive to the extent that they are made without requiring the person's agreement. And the fact that a person may be compliant with a guardianship decision does not stop the decision from being characterised as coercive. The person, for instance, may not have the cognitive or physical ability to object to a guardianship decision to such a degree as to challenge its effectiveness. In addition to this, guardians can be given explicit coercive authority to obtain access to a represented person and to compel compliance with a guardianship decision (*Guardianship and Administration Act 1986* Vic, sections 26 and 27). OPA (2016) obtained 41 orders of this nature in 2015–16, with police attendance required in 13 situations.

It is worth noting that, in addition to its last-resort guardianship role, OPA has safeguarding roles in relation to coercive interventions. OPA has a monitoring role in relation to the restrictive intervention and compulsory treatment provisions under the *Disability Act 2006* Vic (sections 143, 144, 191, 194, 196, 199) and in relation to the *Severe Substance Dependence Treatment Act 2010* Vic (sections 25, 27). OPA also registers notices in relation to non-emergency medical treatment of adults who are unable to consent to such treatment (*Guardianship and Administration Act 1986*, section 42K). From March 2018, OPA will be the automatic decision-maker of last resort for 'significant' medical treatment decisions where no other decision-maker is available (*Medical Treatment Planning and Decisions Act 2016* Vic, section 63).

Some jurisdictions enable guardians to have slightly different, and in some cases, expanded roles. For instance, Queensland's guardianship legislation enables guardians to consent to restrictive interventions (see *Guardianship and*

Administration Act 2000 Qld, section 80ZE). This, in OPA's view, is not ideal (see Williams, Chesterman & Laufer, 2014, especially pp. 655ff).

Critiques of substitute decision-making

International human rights law is increasingly intolerant of substitute decision-making, preferring other approaches that support people with disabilities to make and implement their own decisions. The *Convention on the Rights of Persons with Disabilities* is the exemplar of this approach. Article 12 holds that: 'persons with disabilities enjoy legal capacity on an equal basis with others in all aspects of life' and that:

> all measures that relate to the exercise of legal capacity provide for appropriate and effective safeguards ... Such safeguards shall ensure that measures relating to the exercise of legal capacity respect the rights, will and preferences of the person ... apply for the shortest time possible and are subject to regular review by a competent, independent and impartial authority or judicial body.

The Convention's treaty-monitoring committee, the Committee on the Rights of Persons with Disabilities (2014), has gone so far as to say that:

> States parties' obligation to replace substitute decision-making regimes by supported decision-making requires both the abolition of substitute decision-making regimes and the development of supported decision-making alternatives. The development of supported decision-making systems in parallel with the maintenance of substitute decision-making regimes is not sufficient to comply with article 12 of the Convention.
>
> (par. 28)

This far-reaching statement calls bluntly for the abolition of all substitute decision-making regimes. In Australia, this would involve every state and territory removing key elements of their guardianship, mental health, powers of attorney and medical treatment laws.

While the language of the comment is clear, few people, when pressed, would hold to the view that there is never a place for substitute decision-making. If an unconscious patient in hospital requires a medical decision to be made, but has no family or friends available, or written instructions on file, what should occur? Should medical staff be able to proceed regardless, or should an independent substitute decision-maker be appointed?

Even the strongest critics of guardianship struggle with proposing alternatives to such difficult cases. Michael Bach and Lana Kerzner (2010), for example, discuss the possibility of 'facilitated decision making' in relation to people whose significant disabilities prevent them from acting independently and who are not able to be supported to make decisions. An appointment in these circumstances might be made by the person themselves in an advance document or by an administrative tribunal. The powers of the facilitator, according to this reform idea (Bach & Kerzner, 2010), would be constrained to acting according to the person's previously expressed wishes and in such a way as to improve the person's quality of life. However, in many ways this kind of appointment would be similar to the appointment of a guardian with limited powers.

The Australian Law Reform Commission (ALRC) has considered the view of the Committee on the Rights of Persons with Disabilities and has concluded (ALRC, 2014) that 'some system of appointment of others to act is a necessary human rights backstop' (par. 2.107). In arguing for a continued, albeit limited, place for substitute decision making, the ALRC (2014) drew a distinction between 'the appointment of a person to act' and 'the standard by which the appointee – or substitute – is to act' (par. 2.74). The ALRC took the view 'that the UNCRPD was principally condemning a best interests approach, not a will and preferences approach' (par. 2.96).

Here the ALRC drew a distinction between the bases on which substitute decision-making can occur. A 'best interests' approach is one where the substitute decision-maker determines for themselves what they consider to be in the person's best interests. A 'will and preferences' approach sees the substitute decision-maker's decision being based on what the person themselves would have decided, were they able to do so. This is also known as a 'substituted judgement' approach.

As an example of the changing legal landscape in this regard, Victoria's guardianship legislation currently utilises a 'best interests' approach, even though guardians are required to take 'into account, as far as possible, the wishes of the represented person' (*Guardianship and Administration Act 1986* Vic, section 28). However, the more contemporary *Medical Treatment Planning and Decisions Act 2016* Vic (section 61) adopts a substituted judgement approach.

For the ALRC (2014) any representative decision-making, which should only ever be used as a last resort, should be informed by a substituted judgement approach that prioritises the 'will, preferences and rights of persons' (pars. 2.74, 3.4; see also Law Commission of Ontario, 2015, p. 145). The ALRC (2014) has proposed the adoption of 'national decision-making principles' that would guide reforms to 'Commonwealth, state and territory laws and legal frameworks concerning individual decision-making' (p. 11). The key aims of this reform would be

to ensure that:

- supported decision-making is encouraged;
- representative decision-makers are appointed only as a last resort; and

- the will, preferences and rights of persons direct decisions that affect their lives.

(ALRC, 2014, p. 11)

The ALRC (2014) proposed the use of the terms 'supporter' and 'representative' as the two different kinds of providers of decision-making support (p. 12). It recommended that:

Where a representative is appointed to make decisions for a person who requires decision-making support:

a   The person's will and preferences must be given effect.
b   Where the person's current will and preferences cannot be determined, the representative must give effect to what the person would likely want, based on all the information available, including by consulting with family members, carers and other significant people in their life.
c   If it is not possible to determine what the person would likely want, the representative must act to promote and uphold the person's human rights and act in the way least restrictive of those rights.

It is hard to know in practice what it will mean to 'promote and uphold the person's human rights' if a person's disability is so profound as to make it hard to infer meaningfully what their will and preferences are, or may have been, though the ALRC (2014) has proposed that several rights be considered in coming to this conclusion. The ALRC (2014) proposed that this model be incorporated in multiple Commonwealth legislative schemes, including the *Aged Care Act*, and that it underwrite the review of state and territory guardianship and related laws. The ALRC report is starting to have an impact, with the *My Health Records Act 2012* (Commonwealth) now incorporating a provision requiring representatives to 'give effect to the healthcare recipient's will and preferences, or likely will and preferences' unless 'to do so would pose a serious risk to the healthcare recipient's personal and social wellbeing' (section 7A).

In relationship to guardianship, the key message from the Convention, which the ALRC (2014) has promoted and as I have argued (Chesterman, 2013a), is that the Convention obliges all parties to use guardianship as sparingly as possible and to limit the powers exercised by guardians. This trajectory is welcome and very important, given history's innumerable examples of the presence of disability leading to outrageous human rights abuses, including mass institutionalisation and physical and other abuse. This trajectory is clearly relevant to the reviews of the guardianship laws in force in

Australia, which on the whole are dated. It has informed the reviews of guardianship laws that have been conducted by the Queensland Law Reform Commission (2010) and Victorian Law Reform Commission (VLRC 2012, see also Chesterman 2010, 2013b), and it is central to the New South Wales Law Reform Commission's (2015) current review of guardianship laws. The Australian Law Reform Commission (2014) recommended that all 'state and territory governments should review laws and legal frameworks concerning individual decision-making' (p. 274).

While Australian reform is proceeding, the international human rights movement away from substitute decision-making is occurring at the same time as a competing drive for greater formalism and certainty in relation to future decision-making for people with lifelong significant cognitive impairments. The concerns of ageing carers, and their belief in the authoritative status that guardianship would give them, have prompted some initiatives designed to make the pathway to guardianship easier for parents of people with lifelong disabilities. For instance, the VLRC (2012) made one recommendation (rec. 176) along these lines, and a version of this appeared in a Victorian Bill (Guardianship and Administration Bill 2014, Part 5) that lapsed prior to the 2014 Victorian state election. This kind of development, which would clearly be contrary to Australia's human rights commitments, should be resisted. At the same time, the valid concerns of parents who are lifelong carers should be met in other ways. This could include an enhanced advocacy status for parents of children who have significant cognitive impairments, which could be accompanied by a rebuttable legislated right to be consulted on significant service developments affecting their children (see OPA, 2012).

It is likely Australia's guardianship laws will gradually be reformed in line with recent and current law reform commission reports to make the criteria for the appointment of a guardian narrower, and to prioritise the actual and likely wishes of represented persons over the more paternalistic protection of their 'best interests'. At the same time, guardianship laws will probably continue to exist.

In the next section I examine some of the current reforms that point to alternatives and developments that can obviate the need for guardianship orders.

Alternatives to guardianship

In considering alternatives to guardianship, it is important to recognise that the modern guardianship system was only ever meant to apply to a small group of people in the population who not only had significant cognitive impairments, but whose wellbeing was currently at risk. To put this another way, most people with cognitive impairments don't have guardians: the VLRC commissioned research which suggests the figure is around 2%

(VLRC, 2012). Informal support mechanisms are the norm, and the existence of informal support, usually provided by family carers, continues to offer the most common reason for the avoidance of guardianship orders. Therefore, in identifying alternatives to guardianship, the promotion of informal support options and less restrictive decision-making pathways is the obvious starting point. There will often be no need for a guardianship order if an individual is able to get supportive friends or relatives to assist them to make decisions.

Another 'informal' mechanism by which guardianship can be avoided is through addressing the particular problem that might otherwise give rise to the appointment of the substitute decision-maker. Guardianship is sometimes utilised where no adequate support service is able to be located, or where possible service responses are unable to be accessed. For instance, guardianship can be a response to a situation of abuse of an older person with a cognitive impairment. A typical example here would be a woman who visits a bank and is coerced by her adult son to withdraw a significant amount of money from her account (Chesterman, 2013b). The use of guardianship here can be the result of a range of factors, including the absence of strong evidence of abuse, and the unwillingness of a victim to make a formal complaint. But the use of guardianship in such situations can effectively amount to a strange form of victim-blaming, in which a person's decision-making authority is removed as a result of their experience of crime (see Chesterman, 2016). Alternatives to guardianship might include improved ability and capacity to prosecute perpetrators and better support mechanisms, including effective case management.

In addition to the possibilities given above, there is a range of more formal alternatives to guardianship. As Kanter (2015) points out, 'a variety of quasi-legal alternatives' to guardianship exist, which 'include health care proxies, durable powers of attorney, representation agreements, trust funds, case management services, special needs trusts, and even special bank accounts' (p. 54). I examine some of these, and some others, in the sections below.

Supported decision-making

In addition to improved service provision constituting a means of avoiding guardianship, another key reform imperative is the provision of greater levels of support for the individuals concerned to enable them to make their own decisions. An idea that has developed from the long history of informal support being provided to people with significant disability is captured now by the term 'supported decision-making'. Supported decision-making is seen as a particularly important alternative to substitute decision-making. While substitute decision-making involves a person making a decision for someone else, supported decision-making involves the person themselves making decisions, but with the support of others.

While there have been significant pilot studies in Australia (Browning, Bigby & Douglas, 2014; Carney, 2014), including two involving OPA (Vic) (see Burgen, 2016), and significant calls for law reform (e.g., VLRC, 2012), there has been very little legislative recognition in Australia of supported decision-making. One notable recent exception is Victoria's *Powers of Attorney Act 2014*, which came into force on 1 September 2015. That Act (part 7) enables a principal to appoint a 'supportive attorney'. While the principal retains decision-making authority, the supportive attorney has legal power to obtain information (overcoming privacy restrictions) and can put decisions into effect (aside from those concerning 'significant financial transactions'). Similarly, the *Medical Treatment Planning and Decisions Act 2016* Vic (sections 31 and 32) introduced the role of 'support person', who can be appointed by the patient to assist them in making medical treatment decisions.

This is an area in which further developments are anticipated. For instance, Ireland's *Assisted Decision-Making (Capacity) Act 2015* (Parts 3 and 4) provides new supported decision-making possibilities under the headings of 'assisted decision-making' and 'co-decision-making'.

NDIS nominees

Another alternative to existing substitute decision-making processes is contained in the legislation and rules governing the National Disability Insurance Scheme (NDIS). The scheme, which began in launch sites in 2013 and is gradually being implemented throughout the country, will ultimately result in 'reasonable and necessary supports' being provided to 460,000 people with disability who have 'substantially reduced functional capacity' (*NDIS Act 2013*, sections 3, 24). The NDIS is based on a consumer choice model that will 'enable people with disability to exercise choice and control' in the provision of supports (*NDIS Act* section 3). While this principle is clearly stated, its implementation poses challenges when the person concerned has a significant cognitive impairment. The same can be said of contemporaneous aged care 'consumer choice' changes (see Chesterman, 2014).

More than half of the participants in the NDIS have disabilities that affect decision-making ability (National Disability Insurance Agency, 2016). While the principles underpinning the legislation promote the need for people to be supported in exercising their choices (NDIS Act, section 4), the Act does provide (sections 78 and 86) for substitute decision-making through the appointment by the NDIA of 'plan nominees' who can have substitute decision-making power. In appointing nominees 'regard' must be given to whether anyone has been appointed to make decisions for the person under state or territory guardianship laws (s. 88; see further ALRC, 2014, pp. 147–53).

As a matter of practice, it has been unclear when an NDIS participant or prospective participant might need a nominee to act on their behalf. It has also been unclear when a guardianship application under state or territory laws might be needed in relation to a person's engagement with the NDIS. The agreement between the NDIA and participants about the nature of funded supports has proven not to be (strictly speaking) a contractual process in which an agreement is reached between the NDIA and the participant or their nominee. Rather, the process has involved the NDIA determining, on the basis of discussions with participants and those around them, which supports will be funded. So, while nominees do exist as potential substitute decision-makers, it is unclear how much they will be used as the NDIS rolls out.

Enduring powers of attorney

Tribunal-appointed guardians and NDIS nominees are examples of substitute decision-makers being appointed on a person's behalf. Enduring powers of attorney are legal instruments that enable individuals to appoint their own decision-makers. Powers of attorney are common but their actual usage levels are not known, because there is no general requirement to register them (although some jurisdictions do require registration when land dealings are involved, and Tasmania requires registration of enduring powers of guardianship; see VLRC, 2012).

Advance directives

Another option, which can mean a person does not need to have a guardian appointed for them, can involve the person making their choices clear in advance through completion of an advance care plan or 'living will'. This tends to have most relevance to medical treatment, but there is no reason why advance plans could not incorporate the ability of people to make wishes about non-medical as well as medical treatment matters known in advance. Indeed the VLRC (2012) recommended that Victoria's law be changed to enable people to provide 'binding instructions or advisory instructions about health matters' and 'advisory instructions about personal and lifestyle matters' (p. 221). That recommendation largely came to fruition with the passage of the *Medical Treatment Planning and Decisions Act 2016* Vic (section 6), which enables people to make both binding and advisory health directives.

Conclusion

Adult guardianship laws are likely to continue to be a feature of Australian law, but the criteria for guardianship appointments are likely to be narrowed in years ahead, in line with the trajectory of international human rights law. At the same time, substitute decision-making, when it is permitted, is likely to be required to be exercised on a substituted judgement basis more often. That is, decision-makers will increasingly be required to make decisions that accord with what the person would themselves have wanted to happen, not what the decision-maker considers to be in the person's 'best interests'. While these changes are important, it is equally important that a range of other legal and service reforms occur, such as those briefly articulated above, to ensure that guardianship orders are made only in situations of absolute necessity.

References

Australian Law Reform Commission (2014). *Equality, capacity and disability in Commonwealth laws.* Report 124. Canberra: ALRC.

Bach, M., & Kerzner, L. (2010). *A new paradigm for protecting autonomy and the right to legal capacity.* Toronto, Ontario: Law Commission of Ontario.

Browning, M., Bigby, C., & Douglas, J. (2014). Supported decision making: Understanding how its conceptual link to legal capacity is influencing the development of practice. *Research and Practice in Intellectual and Developmental Disabilities, 34–35.* doi:10.1080/23297018.2014.902726.

Burgen, B. (2016). Reflections on the Victorian Office of the Public Advocate supported decision-making pilot project. *Research and Practice in Intellectual and Developmental Disabilities, 165–181.* doi:10.1080/23297018.2016.1199969.

Carney, T. (2014). Clarifying, operationalising, and evaluating supported decision making models. *Research and Practice in Intellectual and Developmental Disabilities,* doi:10.1080/23297018.2014.902727.

Carney, T., & Tait, D. (1997). *The adult guardianship experiment: Tribunals and popular justice.* Sydney: Federation Press.

Chesterman, J. (2010). The review of Victoria's guardianship legislation: State policy development in an age of human rights. *Australian Journal of Public Administration 69,* 61–65.

Chesterman, J. (2013a). The future of adult guardianship in federal Australia. *Australian Social Work 66:* 26–38.

Chesterman, J. (2013b). *Responding to violence, abuse, exploitation and neglect: Improving our protection of at-risk adults.* Churchill Fellowship report, available via www.churchilltrust.com.au

Chesterman, J. (2014). Modernising adult protection in an age of choice. *Australian Journal of Public Administration 73,* 517–524.

Chesterman, J. (2016). Taking control: Putting older people at the centre of elder abuse response strategies. *Australian Social Work 69(1),* 115–124.

Committee on the Rights of Persons with Disabilities (2014). General comment No. 1, CRPD/C/GC/1.

Kanter, A. S. (2015). Guardianship for young adults with disabilities as a violation of the purpose of the Individuals with Disabilities Education Improvement Act. *Journal of International Aging Law and Policy 8,* 1–67.

Law Commission of Ontario (2015). *Legal capacity, decision-making and guardianship: Interim report.* Toronto, Ontario: Law Commission of Ontario. www.lco-cdo.org/en/capacity-guardianship-interim-report

National Disability Insurance Agency (NDIA) (2016). *11th Quarterly Report to COAG Disability Reform Council.* https://myplace.ndis.gov.au/ndisstorefront/about-us/information-publications-and-reports/quarterly-reports.html

New South Wales Law Reform Commission (2015). *Review of the Guardianship Act 1987*. Sydney: New South Wales Law Reform Commission. www.lawreform.justice. nsw.gov.au/Pages/lrc/lrc_current_projects/Guardianship/Guardianship.aspx

Office of the Public Advocate (Victoria) (2012). *Response to the Victorian Law Reform Commission's Final Report on Guardianship*. Melbourne: Office of the Public Advocate.   www.publicadvocate.vic.gov.au/our-services/publications-forms/research-reports/guardianship/guardianship-law-reform/30-response-to-the-victorian-law-refo rm-commissions-final-report-on-guardianship

Office of the Public Advocate (Victoria) (2015). *Office of the Public Advocate Annual Report 2014–15*. Melbourne: Office of the Public Advocate.

Office of the Public Advocate (Victoria) (2016). *Office of the Public Advocate Annual Report 2015–16*. Melbourne: Office of the Public Advocate.

Queensland Law Reform Commission (2010). *A review of Queensland's guardianship laws: Report*. Vols. 1–4. Brisbane: Queensland Law Reform Commission.

Victorian Law Reform Commission (2012). *Guardianship Final Report*. Melbourne: Victorian Law Reform Commission.

Victorian Civil and Administrative Tribunal (2015). *VCAT Annual Report 2014–2015*. Melbourne: Victorian Civil and Administrative Tribunal.

Williams, M., Chesterman, J., & Laufer, R. (2014). Consent versus scrutiny: Restricting liberties in post-Bournewood Victoria. *Journal of Law and Medicine* 21, 641–660.

Legislation

Assisted Decision-Making (Capacity) Act 2015 (Ireland)
Convention on the Rights of Persons with Disabilities
Disability Act 2006 (Vic)
Guardianship and Administration Act 1986 (Vic)
Guardianship and Administration Act 2000 (Qld)
Guardianship of Adults Act 2016 (NT)
Medical Treatment Planning and Decisions Act 2016 (Vic)
Mental Health Act 2014 (Vic)
My Health Records Act 2012 (Commonwealth)
NDIS Act 2013 (Commonwealth)
Powers of Attorney Act 2014 (Vic)
Severe Substance Dependence Treatment Act 2010 (Vic)

Index

Aboriginal trust accounts 137; *see also* Healthy Welfare Card

academic writing, process of 4

'acceptable' treatments: addiction medicine, ambivalence to involuntary treatment 45–6

Adams, B. 165

Adams, D.L., & Erevelles, N. 100, 101

addiction: behavioural evidence 20; brain disease model of 18–19; brain disease model of, plausibility of 20; choice model of 19–20; compulsory treatment of 23–4; conceptualisations of 123–5, 125–6, 130–31; effectiveness of compulsory treatment of 24; ethicality of coerced treatment of 21, 24–5; models of 18–20, 25n3; neuroimaging studies 19, 20; NSW Standing Committee on Social Issues on compulsory treatments 24; PwC's Indigenous Consulting with Menzies School of Health Research 23; terminology of 25n1; United Nations Office on Drugs and Crime (UNODC) 24, 25; World Health Organization (WHO) 21

addiction medicine, ambivalence to involuntary treatment 44–55; 'acceptable' treatments 45–6; addiction medicine patients, special issues in relation to 50–51; case presentations 46–9; central nervous system (CNS), damage to 49–50; clinically driven involuntary treatments 52; compulsory treatment for dependent patients, observations on 44; constructive case for better way forward 53–4;

correctional services coerced (involuntary) interventions 52; dependent individuals, actions of 48–9; Drug and Alcohol Court Assessment Program (DACAP) in NSW 52; efficacy of involuntary treatment 50–51; employment of involuntary treatment programs 44–5; Inebriates Act (1912), New South Wales 51; interventional approach, clinical support for 54–5; involuntary or mandated treatment programs for those with dependency 52–3; Magistrates Early Referral into Treatment (MERIT) in NSW 52; mandated treatment programs for drug dependence, employment of 44–5; mandated treatment strategies, conditions for use of 53–4; mandated treatment strategies for recovering professionals 52–3; mental health specialty, involuntary treatment in 46; multiple drug use dependency, case of 47; organ damage in drug-using individuals 49–50; proposal for way forward (based on evidence and lack of it) 53–4; rational decision-making about drug use 48; resistance to involuntary treatment 44; severe alcohol use disorder, case of 47–8; treatment outcome literature, evidence from 50

adult guardianship and alternatives 225–34; adult guardianship laws 233–4; advance directives 233; Aged Care Act (Commonwealth) 229; alternatives to guardianship 230–33; Assisted Decision-Making (Capacity)